S0-CFO-000

ATTEMPTING WORK REFORM

Wiley Series On
ORGANIZATIONAL ASSESSMENT AND CHANGE

Series Editors:
Edward E. Lawler III and
Stanley E. Seashore

ATTEMPTING WORK REFORM

The Case of "Parkside" Hospital

MARTIN D. HANLON
*Queens College of the City
University of New York*

DAVID A. NADLER
Delta Consulting Group, Inc.

DEBORAH GLADSTEIN
Dartmouth College

A WILEY-INTERSCIENCE PUBLICATION

JOHN WILEY & SONS

New York • Chichester • Brisbane • Toronto • Singapore

Copyright © 1985 by John Wiley & Sons, Inc.

All rights reserved. Published simultaneously in Canada.

Reproduction or translation of any part of this work
beyond that permitted by Section 107 or 108 of the
1976 United States Copyright Act without the permission
of the copyright owner is unlawful. Requests for
permission or further information should be addressed to
the Permissions Department, John Wiley & Sons, Inc.

This publication is designed to provide accurate and
authoritative information in regard to the subject
matter covered. It is sold with the understanding that
the publisher is not engaged in rendering legal, accounting,
or other professional service. If legal advice or other
expert assistance is required, the services of a competent
professional person should be sought. *From a Declaration
of Principles jointly adopted by a Committee of the
American Bar Association and a Committee of Publishers.*

Library of Congress Cataloging in Publication Data

Hanlon, Martin D.
    Attempting Work Reform

    (Wiley series on organizational assessment and change,
ISSN 0737-7290)
    "A Wiley-Interscience publication."
    Bibliography: p.
    Includes index.
    1. Hospitals—Personnel management. 2. Quality of
work life. 3. Trade-unions—Hospitals. 4. Organizational
change. 5. Organizational effectiveness. 6. Hospitals,
Teaching I. Nadler, David. II. Gladstein, Deborah.
III. Title. IV. Title: "Parkside" Hospital. V. Series.
RA971.35.H37 1985   362.1′1′0683   84-13189
    ISBN 0-471-88766-8

Printed in the United States of America

10   9   8   7   6   5   4   3   2   1

Series Preface

The ORGANIZATIONAL ASSESSMENT AND CHANGE SERIES is concerned with informing and furthering contemporary debate on the effectiveness of work organizations and the quality of life they provide for their members. Of particular relevance is the adaptation of work organizations to changing social aspirations and economic constraints. There has been a phenomenal growth of interest in the quality of work life and productivity in recent years. Issues that not long ago were the quiet concern of a few academics and a few leaders in unions and management have become issues of broader public interest. They have intruded upon broadcast media prime time, lead newspaper and magazine columns, the houses of Congress, and the board rooms of both firms and unions.

A thorough discussion of what organizations should be like and how they can be improved must comprehend many issues. Some are concerned with basic moral and ethical questions—What is the responsibility of an organization to its employees?—What, after all, is a "good job"?—How should it be decided that some might benefit from and others pay for gains in the quality of work life?—Should there be a public policy on the matter? Yet others are concerned with the strategies and tactics of bringing about changes in organizational life, the advocates of alternative approaches being numerous, vocal, and controversial; and still others are concerned with the task of measurement and assessment on grounds that the choices to be made by leaders, the assessment of consequences, and the bargaining of equities must be informed by reliable, comprehensive, and relevant information of kinds not now readily available.

The WILEY SERIES ON ORGANIZATIONAL ASSESSMENT AND CHANGE is concerned with all aspects of the debate on how organizations should be managed, changed, and controlled. It includes books on organizational effectiveness, and the study of organizational changes that represent new approaches to organization design and process. The volumes in the series have in common a concern with work organizations, a focus on change and the dynamics of change, an assumption that diverse social and personal interests need to be taken into account in discussions of organizational effectiveness, and a view that concrete cases and quantitative data are essential ingredients in a lucid debate. As such, these books consider a broad but integrated set of issues and ideas. They are intended to be read by managers, union officials, researchers, consultants, policy makers, students, and others seriously concerned with organizational assessment and change.

EDWARD E. LAWLER, III
STANLEY E. SEASHORE

Los Angeles, California
Ann Arbor, Michigan

Preface

This book describes a quality of work life project that was carried out in a prominent teaching hospital located in a large city in the northeastern United States. The goal of the project at Parkside—the name we have given to the hospital—was to involve management, the hospital's major unions, and external behavioral science consultants in a collaborative effort to improve patient care and the quality of work life of employees. The project spanned a period of nearly four years, from 1974 to 1978. During this time, we were the principal members of an independent research team based in the Columbia University Graduate School of Business that documented the history of the project and assessed its outcomes.

The Parkside project was significant in several respects. First, it was one of the first quality of work life projects in the United States that involved more than one union. Initially, the Parkside QWL project was sponsored by three major unions in the hospital, unions which represented a diverse range of occupations from resident physicians to unskilled service personnel. At the time of the project, union-management collaboration to improve the quality of work life was still a rather novel idea. Apart from a few notable exceptions, such as the United Automobile Workers, American unions were quite wary of becoming involved in projects such as QWL that lay beyond the traditional scope of collective bargaining. Some unions viewed QWL as an explicitly antiunion movement. Other unions accepted the humanistic goals of QWL but questioned whether the emphasis on work place reform would divert attention from organized labor's attempts to improve wages, benefits, job security, and occupational health and safety. In this context of general mistrust toward QWL, bringing together three unions into a collaborative relationship with one another and with management was a notable accomplishment.

Second, the Parkside project was one of the first attempts to apply what might be termed the *QWL collaborative model* to a large medical care organization. Much of the theory and practice of quality of work life interventions and the behavioral science groundwork of QWL have been developed in the context of industrial organizations in the private sector. An important question is whether the types of intervention strategies that have proved effective in private industry are appropriate to complex service organizations—a hospital in this case—where the "product" is saving human life. The Parkside project led us to the general conclusion that while there is an enormous potential for quality of work life improvement in hospitals, there are also an incredible number of ways in which such a project could fail. For its size, no organization rivals a modern tertiary care hospital in complexity. This complexity makes the process of improving quality of work life singularly difficult. In the final chapter of this book we argue that QWL interventions in hosptials are unlikely to succeed if limited to the improvement of interpersonal and intergroup relations; rather, questions of organizational structure must always be a principal focus of a QWL change strategy.

A third notable aspect of the Parkside project was the careful attention given to the documentation of its course and the assessment of its impact on the hospital. Parkside was one of eight demonstration projects initiated through the Michigan Quality of Work Program. The Michigan program involved a specific model of organizational change—based on a collaborative relationship between management and employee unions (all eight project sites were unionized)—and a strong emphasis on an independent and relatively standardized method of project assessment. Parkside and its sister projects afforded a rare opportunity to combine organizational change with scientific research.

In the course of our research activity at Parkside, we relied heavily on the data gathering approach known as *participant observation*. As we will describe in this book, our strategy changed from one that stressed different types of quantitative measurement to one that was better suited to understanding the complexity of a large scale organizational change project. We came to feel that the rapidly growing body of literature devoted to quality of work life has not conveyed successfully the feelings and behavior of participants in QWL projects, nor has this literature addressed the dynamic (and often frustrating) elements of QWL. The years of field work that formed the core of our assessment effort made us very sympathetic to the employees of Parkside and the project consultants as they struggled to improve the workings of a difficult organization. We hope that we have succeeded in preserving some measure of scientific objectivity while making use of the subjective element that is in the best tradition of organization research.

MARTIN D. HANLON
DAVID A. NADLER
DEBORAH GLADSTEIN

New York, New York
New York, New York
Hanover, New Hampshire
October 1984

Acknowledgments

Over the years our research on this project benefited immeasurably from the work of a talented and committed team of graduate assistants at Columbia. To John Cox, Adam Halasi-Kun, Harvery Wallender, Laura Gradford, Deborah Stoll, Ann Matterson, and Janet Handal—many thanks.

We acknowledge the support of James C. Daugherty of the National Center for Health Systems Research, who was the project officer for "Parkside," and Dr. Sumner M. Rosen of Columbia University, who served as outside consultant to HEW on the project. Thanks also to Ted Mills and Nick Bizony of the National Quality of Work Center (now the American Center for the Quality of Working Life).

We are grateful to David Berg of Yale, who was extremely helpful in the role of process consultant during the early stages of the Parkside Project. Phil Mirvis of Boston University contributed many useful ideas and criticisms on earlier drafts of this book. Special thanks goes to Ed Lawler of the University of Southern California, who was so generous in his support throughout the history of the project.

We are indebted to Judith Dumas, who typed the drafts of this book, and to Edward Max Rosen for his research assistance during the preparation of this manuscript.

Unfortunately, considerations of confidentiality prevent us from acknowledging by name the many staff members, managers, and union officials who contributed so much of their time and attention to our project evaluation efforts. We thank them all, especially our friends from Barnard 5.

M.D.H.
D.A.N.
D.G.

xi

Contents

CHAPTER ONE

Introduction

No country devotes more of its resources to medical care than the United States. As a result of a long-term health cost inflation rate more than double that of the economy as a whole, over 10 percent of the U.S. Gross National Product is allocated to the medical industry. Apart from cost issues, the rhetoric of crisis that dominates public discussions of our health care system reflects popular disillusionment with what the medical dollar actually buys. Nowhere is this more evident than in attitudes toward the medical profession. Public admiration for the technical triumphs of modern medicine—organ transplants, *in vitro* fertilization, the well-publicized victories in the "war against cancer," and the revival of the near-dead—is tempered by the belief that greed, not the serving impulse or disinterested professionalism, is at the core of the practice of medicine. As doctors have gained new powers to cure, they have perhaps lost much of their ability to care.

The work of doctoring is carried out in a broad variety of settings in the United States; but the center ring, where medical miracles take place, is the large, tertiary care*, teaching hospital. Popular ambivalence toward the medical profession carries over to the institutions that Paul Starr has termed "awesome citadels of science and bureaucratic order" (1982, p. 145). Far removed from its earlier function as a custodial facility where chronically or terminally ill (and generally poor) people were sent to die, the hospital offers a uniquely modern

---

Primary care refers to ordinary outpatient care provided in a physician's office or clinic. *Secondary care* includes office-based specialized medical services and much of the care provided in hospitals. *Tertiary care* refers to highly complex types of care that often involve the utilization of sophisticated medical technology and that are carried out only within specialized hospitals. Tertiary care services include, for example, open heart surgery, organ transplantation, and radiation therapy (see Mechanic, 1979, p. 350).

1

promise of redemption: that a body grossly neglected by its owner and badly in need of repair can be saved and made whole again.

But it is a promise that doesn't come cheap, and the alarm over the huge costs of high technology hospital care has led to a variety of policy initiatives over the past several years. The sheer number of proposals for controlling hospital costs is an indicator of, as much as anything else, the lack of consensus over what can be done. The sense of help-lessness that pervades discourse on the cost problems seems to grow worse as reports of medical breakthroughs from prestigious hospitals increase.

These contradictions and the feelings of alienation engendered by the practice of medicine and the way in which it is organized are felt deeply by hospital patients. Despite numerous reforms in hospital practice that attempt to humanize patient care—such as living-in arrangements for relatives, the growth of patient advocacy, and more thoughtful scheduling procedures—hospital stays are too often described in terms like *depersonalization, resentment, anger, dependence,* and, above all, *fear.* Many of these feelings are of course due to the problems that lead to hospitalization, but the emotional residues that remain long after discharge are often a function of the difficult institutional environment of the hospital.

Neither are hospitals idyllic places to work. A study carried out by research psychologists at the National Institute for Occupational Safety and Health compared incidence rates of mental health disorders, indexed by community mental health center admissions, among 130 major occupational groups (Colligan, Smith, & Hurrell, 1977). The authors report that six of the twenty-two occupations with the highest rates of mental disorder are hospital or health care related (p. 36). They include: health technologists (the group with the highest admissions rate among the 130 groups), practical nurses, clinical lab technicians, nurse's aides, health aides, and registered nurses.

To understand the roots of these problems, it is necessary to comprehend the formal organizational characteristics of hospitals. For its size, the modern tertiary care hospital is perhaps the most complex type of bureaucratic organization ever created. Hospitals, particularly those located in urban areas, bring together people of vastly different backgrounds, experience, and aptitudes and connect them through an enormously complicated web of roles, groups, and administrative and technical functions. Social scientists have struggled to capture the essence of the modern hospital through descriptive concepts such as "multiple lines of authority" and in a number of field studies of conflicts among staff. In Chapter 3 we present our own analysis of the "nature" of the hospital. We do so with modesty. In a single book, it is difficult to convey how a hospital works, how the unique culture of a hospital shapes attitudes and behaviors, or how the complex systems of the human body are mapped into the array of specialized departments and subdepartments that is the most notable characteristic of giant tertiary care medical centers.

THE HOSPITAL AS A FOCUS OF ORGANIZATIONAL CHANGE

Over the past several years, there have been many proposals for improving the functioning of hospitals. Most can be viewed as attempts to rationalize the hospital, to bring its administrative and financial systems into line with those of other types of bureaucratic organizations. Prescriptions vary, but the general thrust is to extend the effective range of managerial control—often at the expense of the medical staff. Other proposals have given more attention to the political aspects of hospital organization. Here, the emphasis is on accommodating the competing interests of different power centers—physicians, administrators, the board of trustees, the unions, and the community at large—in ways that optimize organizational performance. Both of these approaches—the rationalistic and the political—take the existing hierarchical nature of the hospital as a given. In the parlance of organizational change strategists, they are "top-down" perspectives.

This book describes a significant attempt to improve the workings of a large tertiary care hospital located in a city in the eastern United States that took a very different approach from those described above. In brief, the Parkside Hospital Quality of Work Life Project* was an attempt at organizational reform through a broad program of employee participation. The emphasis was on democratic, "bottom-up" types of change.

The Parkside Project had two overriding goals. One was *to improve the overall functioning of the hospital.* As we describe later, Parkside enjoyed an international reputation for scientific medicine. Through its prestigious medical school†, Parkside is a well-known center of in-

---

*Disguised names for the hospital and all individual participants, with the exception of individuals associated with the Columbia University research team and the Institute for Social Research of the University of Michigan, will be used throughout the book.
†Parkside Hospital, Parkside Medical School, and a separate corporate body that coordinates the functions of the two major entities comprise the Parkside Medical Center.

novative medical education. But common to other large hospitals, many ranked the quality of nursing care at Parkside far below the quality of medical care. Infection rates on in-patient units posed an embarrassing problem. High staff turnover and consequent problems of understaffing, the need to shift or "float" personnel from one unit to another, and the inexperience of newly hired staff, threatened continuity of care. Heavily unionized, the hospital had, by consensus, an extremely poor labor relations climate—one characterized by a highly adversarial relationship between labor and management and by jurisdiction-based conflicts among the unions as well. None of these factors threatened the hospital's medical standing, but there was a widespread feeling that the hospital did not work well, and that this affected the quality of care received by patients.

Parkside also suffered from a reputation for sloppy management. The director of the hospital, who was appointed at about the same time as the quality of work life project began, was mandated to put a large and basically unkempt house in order. In common with many older voluntary hospitals in the 1970s, Parkside was losing money at an alarming rate, and it lacked basic information about the sources of the "fiscal hemorrhage." The hospital's physical plant paralleled in a striking way the overall lack of coherence in the hospital's administrative structure. It is comprised of a jumble of low, medium, and high-rise buildings that reflects the vicissitudes of architectural style and the changing conceptions of hospital function over a span of eight decades. Basically, the hospital just grew. It would be difficult to design a working hospital as crowded, chaotic, or inefficient as Parkside.

The second major goal of the Parkside Project was to *improve quality of working life* in the hospital. Here again, there could be little disagreement over the need for change. We describe the nature of work at Parkside in detail in Chapter 3 and to some extent throughout the book. But it should be noted here that Parkside was an institution that commanded respect but little love from its employees.

In the chapter that follows this Introduction, we will describe the model of work reform—the quality of work life model—on which the Parkside Project was based. We will also describe the crucial differences between the hierarchical forms of authority characteristic of most large medical institutions, including Parkside, and the more democratic, participative organizational style represented by the quality of work life model. In the remainder of this chapter, our purpose is to describe the origins and rationale of the Parkside Quality of Work Life (QWL) Project, to discuss some of the key issues in hospital and organizational reform that were raised by the project, and to present the reader with an overview of the rest of the book.

BACKGROUND

The origins of the Parkside Hospital Project date back to 1972, when the Ford Foundation and the U.S. Department of Commerce provided funding for a major series of organizational change projects intended to improve quality of work life and organizational effectiveness (Seashore, 1983). The Institute for Social Research of the University of Michigan assumed responsibility for creating the theoretical foundation of the project series, known as the Michigan Quality of Work Program, and for developing methods to assess the impact of these projects on host organizations. In some projects, including the one at Parkside, the National Quality of Work Center (later renamed the American Center for Quality of Working Life) took responsibility for locating the sites and negotiating the initial agreements. In all cases, the organizations were unionized and the union or unions at each site became cosponsors of the project. The National Quality of Work Center was an affiliate of the Institute for Social Research, which remained responsible for the research activities connected with each of the projects.

The Parkside Project was the fourth in this series of eight experimental projects. Sites included a coal mine, a large public utility, a food company, and a municipal government. To allow for comparative analysis, most of these projects—including Parkside—had a number of structural characteristics in common. What follows is a description of the essential characteristics of the Parkside Project that apply to the Michigan Quality of Work Program as a whole.

First, as noted, the project was established with the dual objectives of improving the effectiveness of the hospital in meeting the needs of patients (an objective that was eventually generalized to "better management") and improving the quality of work life of employees. Like almost all such QWL projects, tangible gains for both the organization and employees were considered corequisites for success. Implicit here is the assumption that the goal of greater organizational effectiveness is compatible with the goal of improving the day-to-day work lives of employees.

Second, the project was based on the use of behavioral science methods for the achievement of goals. This was consistent with the view of the designers of the Michigan Quality of Work Program—that improvements in quality of work life and organizational effectiveness could be best achieved by focusing on the social system of the hospital as opposed to its financial or technical systems.

Third, the project was designed to be a joint labor-management undertaking: It would be "owned" by both management and the legal collective bargaining representatives of different employee groups in the hospital. As a cooperative project, it would seek changes that would benefit both management and the unions.

Fourth, the project was intended to involve all levels of staff in the process of organizational change. Thus "ownership" would be carried over to the employees themselves, not just to their representatives.

Fifth, the Parkside Project, like all other Michigan Program projects, was externally funded. This was deemed necessary because at the time most unions took a skeptical if not hostile position toward such projects. Also, most managements were reluctant to appropriate funds for projects over which they had limited control. The Parkside Project was funded by the Health Services Administration of the U.S. Department of Health, Education & Welfare.

Sixth, the project design called for the use of an outside behavioral science consultant team. Funded by the external grant source, the consultants were expected to view the entire hospital system—unions included—as the client, rather than any single group, faction, or individual.

Seventh, provision was made for an independent assessment of the project by a university-based research team, which was also funded by the external grant source. The research team was to work separately from the consultants and was charged with the description, documentation, and ultimate assessment of project activities.

The authors of this book served as the principal members of the research team over the four-year course of the project. Our role involved intensive on-site observation of major project activities and the collection of data intended to measure the impact of the various project activities on hospital functioning and on quality of work life. Our goals were to provide both a documentary record and an evaluative analysis of the project as a whole, as well as to offer direction for future research and practice.

ISSUES RAISED BY THE PROJECT

In 1973, when the possibility of a QWL project was first proposed to the president of the largest union in the hospital and to hospital management, the QWL movement had limited support. In the same year, General Motors and the GM Department of the United Automobile Workers signed an agreement that launched this country's first corporatewide QWL program. But most union leaders were hesitant to follow the lead of the UAW's Irving Bluestone into cooperative ventures with management and into issues like job satisfaction and expanding the worker's "say" in shop-floor decision making. In the very beginning, the payoffs were uncertain, the dangers of collaboration seemed great, and the formal apparatus of collective bargaining and its basically adversarial nature did not seem well suited to the diffuse, humanistic goals of QWL.

But at least in industrial settings, where most of the new forms of work and organizational experimentation that go under the heading of quality of work life were being carried out, the nature of the work process was generally clear, as were the *potential* benefits of QWL. Taking the quality of work life programs in the automobile industry as a case in point, the gains derived from the more serious QWL efforts were tangible and measurable—fewer production defects, lower absenteeism, fewer grievances, and because of higher quality production, greater job security for employees (see Katz, Kochan, & Gobeille, 1983). From a labor relations perspective, tangible results that benefit both sides—the vaunted "win-win" situation—strengthen the positions of both labor and management and increase the willingness to try out even more innovative ideas. Over the past few years, QWL programs have become a centerpiece of what some experts have called "the new industrial relations" (see Kochan & McKersie, 1983) and have moved from being a peripheral, personnel office issue to becoming, in some cases, an important element in corporate strategic planning (Hanlon, 1985).

But would a QWL program work in a complex tertiary care urban hospital? In the initial meetings that preceded the start of the Parkside Project, representatives of both management and labor expressed the uneasy feeling that "A hospital is different. It may work in a factory but we don't make widgets here." It became clear that most had difficulty comprehending the hospital as an organization, let alone thinking audaciously of how to change it. As researchers, we also had no firm sense of whether or not a model of change derived from manufacturing organizations would work in this most complicated form of service organization.

Hospitals *are* different. In his masterful social history of the development of the medical profession and the health care industry in the United States, Paul Starr describes hospitals as "incompletely integrated . . . a case of blocked institutional development" (1982, p. 179). The hospital is always the exceptional case in theories of organizational structure and behavior, the source of the most interesting but difficult anomalies. To note one example that affected the course of the Parkside Project: A tremendous amount of hospital work is generated by the orders and practices of attending physicians, who, properly speaking, are neither employees of the hospital nor a division of management. It was difficult to accommodate attending physicians within the framework of the labor-management change model. In Chapter 3 we examine the peculiar organizational characteristics of the hospital that make it so difficult to understand and, as we shall later see, to change.

There also appeared to be a fundamental conflict between the democratic, participative ethos of QWL and the hierarchical, quasi-military work relations characteristic of the hospital. At Parkside, work gets done through long chains of command. In patient care areas, orders flow downward from doctors to nurses to nonprofessional staff. Status distinctions are salient and maintained strongly. It was difficult to imagine senior physicians and housekeeping personnel meeting to discuss "shop floor" problems of common concern. Thus apart from our concerns about organizational structure, we questioned whether the authoritarian culture of the hospital would allow for democratic change.

Another issue raised by Parkside is the feasibility of carrying out rigorous research on a large scale program of work reform within a complex, dynamic organization. Field research in organizations is inherently problematic. Moreover, field experiments such as Parkside represent perhaps the most risky and uncertain of field research ventures (Seashore, 1964; Cook & Campbell, 1983). When the consultant and researcher roles are separated, a new set of problems and concerns enter the picture. Conflicts between the needs of the action elements of the project and the demands of valid research design present problems and dilemmas for the researcher (Lawler, Nadler, & Cammann, 1980; Lawler, Nadler, & Mirvis, 1983; Seashore & Mirvis, 1983). The basic question is: How can research be designed and implemented to generate valid data in such a setting?

PLAN OF THE BOOK

The chapters in this book fall into five major groupings of one or more chapters each. First are this introductory chapter and Chapter 2, which present the QWL invervention design. In Chapter 2 we describe the theoretical basis of the project, drawing on the literature of organizational development, labor relations, and quality of work life. Then we delineate the structural model used in the Parkside Quality of Work Life Project. Finally, we present the specific questions that guided the research component of the project.

Second, Chapter 3 describes Parkside Hospital during the 1974–75 start-up period. This chapter includes a brief history of the hospital and of the three major employee unions that were involved in the project. The chapter also includes descriptions of the working environment within the hospital, labor-management relations, and the types of role conflicts that became the focus of several of the project activities. We also describe the patient care (nursing) unit that provided the focus of the project.

Third, Chapters 4–8 provide a detailed history of the Parkside Quality of Work Life Project. Each of the chapters covers a major phase in the development of the project. The five chapters are preceded by a chronological overview of the entire project, from the early negotiations between management and the unions to the Columbia research team's final assessment work.

Fourth, Chapters 9 and 10 assess the Parkside Project. In Chapter 9 we describe the research strategy that was used to document the project and assess its impact on the hospital. We then present the different data collection methods and instruments used in the course of the project. We also discuss some of the critical issues and problems inherent in QWL research. In Chapter 10 the assessment results are presented.

Fifth, in the last chapter of the book, we focus on the limits of quality of work life reform in large and complex medical care settings.

CHAPTER TWO

The Quality of Work Life Intervention Design

The Parkside Project was based on an approach to organizational change that is generally referred to as quality of work life (QWL) or employee involvement. We note in Chapter 1 that most QWL programs have a dual mandate: to improve the effectiveness or productivity of an organization and to improve the work life of employees. In this chapter we describe briefly the characteristic values and organizational practices of QWL. We then examine the theoretical origins and the structure of the specific QWL intervention design that was used at Parkside.

WHAT IS QWL?

The essence of QWL is expansion of employee participation in the decision-making processes of an organization and development of better communication among employees, managers, and union representatives. Most QWL programs are characterized by voluntary participation—at least officially—and are generally limited to work place concerns that lie beyond the normal scope of collective bargaining. Wages, hours of employment, disciplinary procedures, and other contractual matters are usually excluded deliberately from consideration. Apart from the loosely defined goal of greater employee participation, most QWL programs eschew specific objectives. Indeed, QWL advocates often emphasize that it is a process—not something that can be defined in terms of a bound program or project.

Changes that result from QWL range from superficial improvements in the work environment, such as a new paint job in the cafe-

11

teria or housekeeping improvements, to radical efforts to restructure the work process. Many programs emphasize employee training and cover areas such as supervisor-employee relationships, assertiveness training, the design of work groups, and dealing with interpersonal conflicts.

Beginning in the 1970s, several U.S. corporations have designed new production facilities that are based on QWL or "high involvement" principles (Perkins, Nieva, & Lawler, 1983). Such plants, most of which are not unionized, represent the fullest development of QWL as a work place philosophy. Many such plants include features like direct employee involvement in personnel selection, minimal status distinctions between employees and management (typified by a common parking lot and the one-class cafeteria), the elimination of assembly lines through the use of autonomous work groups that are responsible for major subassembly operations, flexible job assignments, and a heavy emphasis on training and career development (see Perkins, Nieva, & Lawler, 1983, Chapter 1).

Most of the published and unpublished reports of high-involvement organizations claim superiority over plants that are designed, staffed, and managed according to traditional practices, although supporting data have limited scientific validity. Still, the weight of the evidence suggests that organizations that are designed from the QWL perspective—by increasing the psychological rewards to employees, by fostering a climate nurturant of innovation, and by maximizing the utilization of available skills—can achieve substantial productivity advantages.

Keeping such organizations going is another matter. The long-term viability of these new, more democratic organizational forms is still an open question. Factors such as changes in key personnel (Walton, 1977) or economic pressures (Perkins, Nieva, & Lawler, 1983) can weaken or destroy the commitment to work innovation and internal democracy that is an essential element of successful QWL-style plants.

The fragile nature of QWL is even more apparent in the case of programs initiated within existing work places. The culture of QWL is often sharply at odds with that of hierarchical, bureaucratic work organizations. Contrast, if you will, a typical quality of work life employee meeting in which everyone—regardless of background or rank—has an equal right to express an opinion, make a criticism, or suggest changes in work procedures with the normal chain-of-command form of organizational decision making. Humanizing a bureaucracy is no easy task, particularly when the focus of change is not specific or easily defined (for example, when adaptions must be made when a new machine is introduced). Humanization demands a radical shift in how people relate to, think about, and work with one another. Institution-alizing change is a major cause for concern in QWL programs that have been carried out in existing organizations as much as it is in pro-grams within new organizations (see Goodman & Dean, 1982). Even in work places that are highly receptive to quality of work life improve-ment (or should be on the basis of existing problems), the counterforces against sustained work life reforms are incredibly strong. As we shall see, nowhere is this more the case than in the modern tertiary care hospital. In the next chapter we examine the question of the fit be-tween the values and practices of the QWL approach and the organizational characteristics of the hospital. First, however, we shall describe the origins of the QWL intervention design used at Parkside.

THE THEORETICAL AND PRACTICAL ORIGINS OF THE QUALITY OF WORK INTERVENTION DESIGN

As noted in Chapter 1, Parkside Hospital was one of a series of project sites of the Michigan Quality of Work Program carried out at the Insti-tute for Social Research (ISR) of the University of Michigan. The ini-tial contact with the management of the hospital and with the three major employee unions was made by a staff member of the ISR-affiliated National Quality of Work Center (now the American Center for the Quality of Working Life). The staff member remained actively involved in the project through its formative period.

The intervention design that has been used in the Quality of Work Program projects, including the one at Parkside, has its origins in three different sources. One is the theory and practice of organization development. Another is the development of approaches for conflict resolution, particularly union-management conflict. These approaches can be subsumed under the heading of "integrative bargaining" (Walton & McKersie, 1965). A third source is the increasing attention being given to the quality of work life of people working in formal or-ganizations. All three sources can be seen as antecedents of the QWL intervention design (see Figure 2.1). Each will therefore be discussed, and their implications for the QWL intervention design identified.

Organizational Development

The field of organizational development seeks to improve organiza-tional effectiveness through the application of knowledge and technologies from the behavioral sciences, particularly in the areas of group and organizational behavior (Beckhard, 1969; Bennis, 1969;

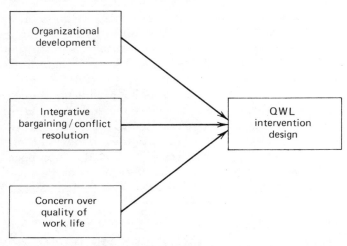

Figure 2.1.   Antecedents of the QWL intervention design.

French & Bell, 1978). The research contribution of organizational development lies in increasing the understanding of how problems can be solved in real settings.

The roots of organizational development go back to a number of very specific insights (French & Bell, 1978). One concerned the importance of process (see Schein, 1969). From the late 1940s, organizational researchers and practitioners became aware of how processes of interpersonal interactions could affect the outcome of those interactions. The implication was that the examination of process could lead to improvement of the effectiveness of individuals, small groups, and even entire organizations. One aspect of process was given particular attention—participation. Early studies (for example, Coch & French, 1948) demonstrated the value of having people participate in making and implementing decisions that affect them (see Vroom, 1964).

A second precursor of organizational development was action research (Sashkin et al., 1973). Here, scientific data collection and analysis methods are applied to the solution of concrete problems. A typical method of action research is survey feedback (see Bowers & Franklin, 1977; Nadler, 1977). Survey data are collected in organizations and fed back to employees for use in problem identification and in problem solving through work sessions.

Over the last three decades, the focus of process-and-action research work moved from the individual to the group level and then from the group to the organizational level of analysis (Katz & Kahn, 1966). Another change has been the shift in emphasis from solely interpersonal process toward a view of process that includes technical and structural concerns as well (Friedlander & Brown, 1974).

While there is great concern about what organizational development actually is and what directions it may take (see Burke, 1976; 1978), several aspects of the practice and theory of organizational development that were drawn on to construct the QWL intervention design can be identified. First, the QWL intervention design makes use primarily of behavioral science techniques and concepts. Second, the major focus of the design is on the system of organizational behavior rather than on the technical, financial, or other types of systems within an organization. Third, the design emphasizes a multiple change approach. Fourth, it is built on basic action research concepts. In particular, the design assumes that diagnosis of a system's problems should precede the prescription or implementation of remedial action. Fifth, the QWL Design incorporates the role of a consultant drawn from outside the target organization who works with organizational members to help create change. Finally, the design includes the use of participative approaches. Those to be affected by changes (or representatives of those affected) are involved in the diagnosis of problems and in the planning and implementation of change.

It is therefore evident that the QWL intervention design reflects many of the values, methods, and technologies of traditional organization development.

Integrative Bargaining

Labor unions are an important element in many work places. The union, empowered to bargain with management over wages, salaries, hours, and conditions of employment, functions as the legal representative of workers. It is reasonable to assume that unions would have a stake in any attempts to change patterns of organizational behavior or efforts to improve the working life of individual employees. The theory and practice of organizational development largely ignored the existence of unions for some time (see Kochan & Dyer, 1976). With a few notable exceptions (Blake, Mouton, & Sloma, 1965; Lewicki & Alderfer, 1973), little or no attention was given to the potential role of unions in facilitating change, resisting change, or being the targets of change.

On the other hand, those who have studied the labor movement have noted that unions and management have at times been able to work together effectively to deal with organizational issues of common concern (see Lesieur, 1957; Walton & McKersie, 1965). This work on labor-management cooperation was another contributing factor to the development of the QWL intervention design. All eight of the original Michigan Quality of Work Program sites included a joint labor-management committee that included representatives from the union or unions at each site. Since then, joint QWL projects have become a major new element in U.S. labor relations (Siegel & Weinberg, 1982), and unions have become much more willing to enter into collaborative programs with management. There are now several national QWL programs cosponsored by a number of major unions, including the United Automobile Workers, the Communications Workers of America, the Steelworkers of America, and the National Association of Letter Carriers. But the Parkside project was initiated during the experimental phase of this development when union mistrust of QWL ran high.

The collective bargaining system in the United States is multidimensional. On the one hand, labor and management clearly have opposing and mutually exclusive interests. On the other, in many areas labor and management have similar goals and thus similar interests. One example might be that of safety, where both parties may have an interest in maintaining a safe working environment.

The well-known work of Walton & McKersie (1965) illustrates the multidimensional nature of collective bargaining relationships. They identify two very different types of bargaining processes in which labor and management engage. The first is termed *"distributive bargaining."* This is the classical zero-sum game situation typically identified with collective bargaining. A fixed "pie" of resources is available, and the bargaining process is one of determining how much of the pie will go to each party. Under such conditions, the only way that one side can increase its resources is to decrease the resources of the other. The bargaining process thus becomes one of proposals, accommodations, threats, and so on, with a recourse to punitive action (strikes or lockouts) if no acceptable distribution agreement is reached.

The second type of bargaining identified by Walton & McKersie, termed, *"integrative bargaining,"* is possible when the objectives of the two parties do not fundamentally conflict (such as in the example of safety mentioned earlier.) Integrative bargaining entails a cooperative problem-solving process in which labor and management work together to identify solutions that will benefit both parties. The result, then, is not the distribution of a fixed set of resources, but the identification of actions that will create value and benefits for both sides.

The Walton and McKersie work was pioneering in that it identified some conditions for creative and constructive conflict resolution. Their approach is consistent with the work of other conflict theorists such as

Follett (Fox & Urwick, 1973) and Deutsch (1973), and it has spurred the development and refinement of conflict resolution models (see Walton, 1969; Filley, 1975; Likert & Likert, 1976; Thomas, 1983.)

As with organizational development, the integrative bargaining and conflict resolution perspective was a source in the development of the QWL intervention design. First, this perspective introduced the idea that labor and management have common interests in the work setting and that those interests (such as quality of work life) might be the focus for cooperative problem solving. Second, previous empirical work in conflict resolution indicated that it is possible to conduct integrative bargaining within the general context of collective bargaining. Third, the perspective suggested that a specific structure for the process of integrative bargaining should be established, a mechanism which would differentiate the integrative and distributive aspects of the labor-management relationship. In many QWL projects, a joint union-management steering committee provides this mechanism.

Concerns about Quality of Work Life

A third source that influenced the development of the QWL intervention design was the growing concern during the early 1970s with the quality of work life in organizations. Traditionally, organizational behavior had focused on factors such as motivation (see Lawler, 1973; Campbell, 1983) and satisfaction (Locke, 1983). Starting in the 1960s and through the 1970s, there developed an awareness of a larger range of issues concerning the consequences of work for individuals.

Much of this new emphasis centered on the consequences for the employee as an individual, rather than as a contributor to organizational effectiveness. Early examples include work in industrial mental health (Kornhauser, 1965; Levinson, Price, Munded, Mandl, & Solley, 1966). There was similar work on the causes and consequences of job stress (Kahn et al., 1964).

The focus on individuals was reinforced in the late 1960s and early 1970s by the attention paid to worker attitudes in the popular press and to some extent in academic circles (U.S. Department of Health, Education & Welfare, 1973). Similarly, many began to define a scope of variables that related to the work place, its characteristics, and its impact on individuals (see for example, Warr & Wall, 1976).

These different streams began to converge in a concern for what came to be called the "Quality of Work Life" (see Davis & Cherns, 1975; Cummings & Molloy, 1977; Hackman & Suttle, 1977). Quality of Work Life is a broad term that includes aspects of the work environ-

Table 2.1.   Influences on the QWL Intervention Design

From Organizational Development	From Integrative Bargaining	Concern About Quality of Work Life (QWL)
Use of behavioral science concepts and technologies	Labor and management do have common interests	A focus on the impact of the workplace on the individual
Focus on system of organizational behavior	Integrative bargaining is possible	A focus on a broad range of aspects of the work environment
Use of other research methods	Need to create a structure to do integrative bargaining	
Consultant's role Participative approaches		

ment (such as conditions of work, job design, participation, and work group functioning), the consequences of the work environment for individuals (such as job satisfaction, stress, mental health, and dysfunctional behaviors), and the methods and technologies for changing the work environment (participative strategies, joint labor-management committees, new plant designs and so on).

The emergence of the Quality of Work Life perspective was a major influence on the QWL intervention design. Specifically, this perspective implied a need to focus on the impact of work and organizational processes on the individual as well as on the organization. A second implication was the need to broaden the focus of activities to include such matters as work design, autonomous group functioning, and so on.

The QWL intervention design can be represented as the convergence of the three sources discussed earlier (see Table 2.1). While this approach has been used widely (see Duckles, Duckles, Drexler & Lawler, 1977; & Maccoby, 1977; and Nadler, 1978), it is just one of a number of possible approaches to changing organizations and the quality of work life.

THE STRUCTURE OF THE QUALITY OF WORK LIFE INTERVENTION DESIGN

The core of the QWL intervention design involves the development of a structure composed of three major parties: a quality of work committee, a consultant or consultant team, and a research team (see Figure 2.2). In this section each of these parties will be described.

The Quality of Work Committee

The collective bargaining literature suggested the need for a specific forum and structure for the integrative bargaining process. The organizational development literature suggested that people in the organization involved must participate in the action research process of diagnosis and intervention if this process is to be successful.

These needs led to the idea of forming a group that would serve as the "client" of the quality of work intervention. It would be a new structure outside of the existing hierarchy and would include representatives of the organization's major groups that had a possible interest in quality of work life and organization change. This design drew upon concepts that relate to the formation of collateral groups for implementing change (Zand, 1974) and the involvement of representatives in a group-client situation (Alderfer, 1977).

In most of the settings that were part of the QWL program, the quality of work committee was to be essentially a joint labor-management

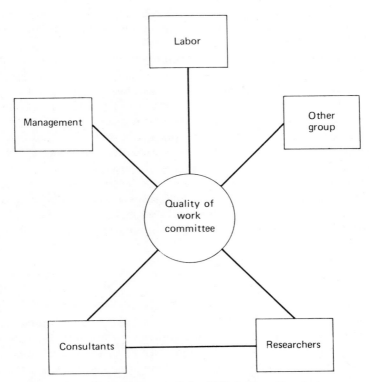

Figure 2.2.   Basic elements of the QWL intervention design.

panel. The committee would include representatives of the management of the parent organization and the particular site (i.e., factory, division, etc.) of the project as well as representatives of the union or unions at that site. In some cases the QWL committee also would include representatives of other employee groups not formally represented by a labor union. Committee decisions were usually to be made by consensus rather than by the potentially more divisive method of voting (see Drexler & Lawler, 1977).

The quality of work committee was established to perform a variety of functions. First, it was to act as a singular client for the consultant, thus helping the consultant to focus and coordinate the needs of the multiple constituencies represented in the project. The dynamics of managing relationships with at least three (and perhaps more) clients can be overwhelming. The committee was to serve as an essential focal point of contact between the consultant and the various groups within the organization.

Second, the committee should serve a representative function. Its existence is meant to ensure that different groups' interests will be reflected in the project activities. It is a safety valve. If problems arise, each group knows that there is a forum where they can be raised, discussed, and resolved.

Third, it should perform a coordinating function. It should manage the project by ensuring the exchange of information, the direction of effort, and the gathering of needed resources at appropriate locations. Typically, a project may involve a variety of activities or, as referred to herein, subprojects. The committee is the place where these activities are linked together, given direction, evaluated, and modified.

Finally, the committee can provide strategic support for the QWL project. By virtue of its membership, it potentially can make things happen. For example, union representatives on the committee might make sure that shop stewards or delegates understand and help in project work; management representatives might arrange for release time or replacement personnel to enable employees to attend project meetings, and so on.

Consultants

The experiences of practitioners in organizational development and conflict resolution indicated that a third party may often be an essential element for making changes and resolving conflicts between two parties. In the Quality of Work Life intervention design, the consultant plays the third party role. He or she is charged with being a change agent (Bennis, 1966) or someone who is primarily concerned with aiding the process of organizational diagnosis and improvement. He or she is frequently less concerned with the content of the change than with the process of change—he or she makes sure that valid information is generated, that participants are able to make free choices about changes and future directions, and that people in the organization develop a commitment to new structures and organizational forms (Argyris, 1970). Thus his or her primary obligation concerns how changes are made, how labor and management work together, and how quality of work life is improved (Schein, 1969).

The kinds of consultant skills necessary for working within the QWL intervention design are those related to the above-stated responsibilities. The consultant needs to draw on concepts, technologies, and skills from the behavioral sciences, particularly in the areas of small group functioning, interpersonal relations, and organizational behavior. The consultant also needs to be someone who, by virtue of credentials, experience, reputation, and interactional style, will be credible in the particular client system in which he or she will work.

Finally, the consultant needs to have an appropriate set of experiences in working with labor unions.

The specific tasks of the consultant in the Quality of Work Life intervention design come under several headings. First, the consultant is responsible for assisting the quality of work committee in identifying goals, pinpointing target areas or issues of change, developing approaches for change, and so on. In helping the committee to work effectively, the consultant must also aid in bringing to the surface and dealing with the inevitable conflicts that will arise among the different parties. Second, the consultant should bring to the project some technical skills in the diagnosis of organizational problems and the formulation of intervention strategies to improve organizational functioning and the quality of work life. The consultant therefore should have a model of organizational functioning and effectiveness, competence in data collection tools and technologies, and experience in doing organizational diagnosis. He or she should also have knowledge and competence in a range of organizational interventions (such as job design, team building, survey feedback, organization design, and training). Third, the consultant is responsible for helping the committee to become a stable and lasting institution for the management of change and the resolution of differences. The quality of work committee represents an opportunity to bring about the institutionalization of change processes. But this can happen only if the committee itself develops processes supportive of its perpetuation, adaptation, and growth.

Researchers

The third major element of the Quality of Work Life intervention design is the research team. There have been two major schools of thought regarding how to structure assessment of change projects in the field. One approach argues for combining the research and consultation roles (see Argyris, 1970). This approach has obvious logistical advantages, and its proponents state that other structural arrangements may lead to intergroup conflict between the researchers and the consultants. The proponents of this approach also contend that if the two perspectives (those of science and of practice) are not integrated, the data generated are less valid than if they are. The alternative view calls for the separation of the research and consultation (Barnes, 1967; Gordon & Morse, 1975; Lawler, 1975). Its proponents argue that when the roles are combined, biases of measurement, analysis, and reporting occur because the researcher cannot be objective about the project. Moreover, they contend the consultation demands will typically override the research demands, thus compromising the validity of the research.

The weight of the empirical evidence appeared to support the latter position; it was decided to use a separate consultation and research approach for the Quality of Work Life intervention design. The research team would be completely separate from the consulting team, and the researchers would be charged with both documenting and evaluating the project as a whole.

An important objective of the research components of all of the Michigan Quality of Work Program projects was to provide some standardized approaches, technologies, and instrumentation for evaluation across a broad range of projects (Lawler, Nadler, & Mirvis, 1983; Seashore, 1983). Uniform methods were developed for use across different projects. They called for the use of standardized technologies—involving multiple measurement modes (questionnaires, interviews, observation, and analysis of secondary data sources)—modified to reflect the specific characteristics of each site and the issues which might emerge during the course of each quality of work life project.

The Total Design

The total design—including the quality of work life committee, the consultants, and the researchers—was created to initiate, implement, evaluate, and disseminate (if appropriate) projects and approaches for improving quality of work life and organizational effectiveness in the host organization. By intent, the structure brought together key power figures and provided the means for taking actions beyond the authority of any single individual, group, or policy-making body. The design provided a mechanism for the diffusion of change and a structure for institutionalizing the quality of work efforts within the ongoing organizational activities. It established a forum for collaboration between different parties and set up a structure of consultants and researchers intended to promote true organizational learning (Argyris & Schon, 1978).

CHAPTER THREE

The Setting of the Quality of Work Life Project

Parkside Hospital

In this chapter, we describe Parkside Hospital in 1975, at the beginning of the quality of work life project. We present the reader with an overview of Parkside as an organization and a description of relations between different employee groups in the hospital. Further on we assess the receptivity of Parkside to a quality of work life project in terms of the QWL model presented in the last chapter. We present our assessment methodology in Chapter 9, but it is important to note here that our description of Parkside at the time of the project is based on more than three years of on-site participant observation, interviews with almost all of the principal figures in the QWL project, and various types of information and data obtained from sources within the hospital.

DESCRIPTION OF PARKSIDE HOSPITAL

Parkside Hospital is a large voluntary (that is, privately endowed—not-for-profit) teaching hospital located in a large city in the eastern United States.

Parkside was founded as a sectarian hospital in the middle of the last century. Around 1900, Parkside acquired its present site, and within a few years, four patient care pavilions were constructed. All remain in use. Like its physical plant, the hospital's reputation has grown steadily to the point where it is now one of the most prestigious hospitals in a city that boasts some of the finest medical care facilities in the world.

The Parkside Medical Center complex straddles a sharp urban ecological boundary that separates an affluent, largely white neighborhood from some of the city's poorest and largely black and Hispanic neighborhoods. The high density housing surrounding the hospital, which includes a substantial amount of high-rise public housing, limits expansion beyond the present site. In common with many urban hospitals, Parkside's capital improvement plans have brought the institution into conflict with the local community, which fears the hospital's encroachment into the neighborhood.

Parkside's emergency entrance is located at the back end of the hospital, separate from its medical and surgical pavilions. The emergency room and an adjacent ambulatory care clinic are used primarily by residents of the surrounding low income neighborhoods. Like all voluntary hospitals in the city, Parkside never refuses emergency treatment to anyone in need, regardless of ability to pay, although the police and the municipal ambulance service deliver most emergency cases to a nearby city-owned hospital. Apart from emergency cases and clinic referrals, admission to Parkside's in-patient units is through its large attending or affiliated medical staff. Parkside's per diem rates are similar to those of the other major teaching hospitals in the city. In 1975, at the time the Parkside Quality of Work Life Project was initiated, the basic rate for a semi-private (usually four-person) room was $225 a day. At present, the basic rate is in excess of $350 a day.

Like many large urban voluntary hospitals, Parkside has, over the years, lost much of its earlier exclusiveness. The hospital's excellent medical reputation assures a steady upper middle class and upper class clientele, but well over half of the hospital's 1200 beds are occupied by Medicaid and Medicare patients. Some of Parkside's medical and surgical units remain selective, and in these settings, the ratio of private attending physicians to house staff physicians is much higher than in the rest of the hospital, and patient amenities are greater. But differences in the quality of patient care should not be overemphasized. The poor are not shunted away to back wards, nor do the rich enjoy a level of comfort and service found in newer, more exclusive private hospitals. The place has a slightly worn, no-nonsense, utilitarian atmosphere—one that conveys the sense that the hospital's mission is to repair bodies, not provide a relaxing break from everyday life.

Hospital Management

In common with most large teaching hospitals, Parkside has an exceedingly complex leadership structure—one based on the usual triumvirate of a board of trustees, physicians, and professional administrators.

The board of trustees is composed largely of prominent figures in law, medicine, banking and finance, and business. The board has an important influence on the hospital's strategic planning, high-level personnel decisions, and important policy matters (the chairman of the board's concern for the quality of patient care provided an impetus for management support for the quality of work life project), but it is not involved in the actual running of the hospital. This is the province of the physicians and the professional administrators who comprise two highly differentiated hierarchies that coexist in an ambiguous, often conflicting relationship.

Medical authority is shared (with much contention) by several types of physicians. These include: nonpracticing physicians who are full-time administrators; practicing physicians who are also department directors or head a geographically-based function; and the professorial staff of Parkside Medical School, including many doctors who have substantial administrative responsibilities within the hospital. There are also more than 1000 attending physicians affiliated with Parkside. "Attendings," as they are called, are usually not part of the formal medical hierarchy, but they carry substantial influence. Much has been written about the problematic role of the attending physician within the hospital, a role that is illustrated in Goldsmith's operating room description:

> The procedure is performed by a surgeon, probably a white male who is a private practitioner and is billing the patient privately for the procedure. The operating room clothes he wears, the instruments he uses, the facility and other supplies all belong to the hospital. An anesthesiologist, who is also billing the patient privately, is likewise a private entrepreneur who utilizes hospital-owned equipment, which is likely to have been purchased at his request. [1981, p. 102]

There are few parallels to attending physicians in other types of bureaucratic organizations. The origins of this anomalous role go back to the formative era in the development of the modern hospital, a period that Starr dates from 1870 to 1910 (Starr, 1982). The expansion of hospital admitting privileges to large numbers of local physicians occurred after 1900, when rising costs driven by the increasing technological complexity and division of labor in hospitals compelled administrators to tap the abilities of private doctors as income producers. The power of physicians relative to that of hospital trustees increased significantly during this period. A representative case occurred in 1897, when the trustees of Boston City Hospital lost the privilege of admitting patients (Starr, 1982, p. 161). By the end of the first decade of this century, physicians ran the show. And as a measure of its power, the medical profession was able to preserve the entrepreneurial, fee-for-service model within the bureaucratic framework of the hospital—hence, the telling image of the hospital as the "doctor's workshop."

The presence of large numbers of powerful professionals who are under few bureaucratic controls makes the task of coordinating the complex work of modern hospitals enormously difficult and increases the need for a large administration. As Robert Guest describes the problem: "The doctor was and is still officially 'a guest' of the open staff hospital. Many of today's most difficult policy questions facing governing boards, administrators, and doctors revolve around this central fact" (1972, p. 286).

The professional administrative hierarchy at Parkside is headed by the director of the hospital who holds a master's degree in Business Administration. Parkside's management structure has undergone several changes since the quality of work life project began in 1975; but at that time, the locus of administrative authority was the hospital's senior management group, which included the director and the heads of financial affairs, development, clinical services, planning and management information systems, support services, labor relations, and nursing. Moreover, each of the hospital's departments (for example, radiology or psychiatry) has an administrative director who shares management responsibilities with the chief physician who is department director.

Beginning with Perrow's (1963) discussion of the changing locus of authority in the development of the modern hospital—from trustees to physicians to professional administrators—organizational researchers have anticipated the day when hospitals will function much like other complex bureaucracies, headed by managers who manage. At Parkside at least, this day remains in the distant future. While the director of the hospital wields considerable influence in all areas of hospital policy—save for areas of decision making that are strictly medical in nature—managers below him have little effective control over the behavior of full-time physician administrators, particularly the department chiefs, and even less over the vast army of attendings. It is common for the professional administrators—armed with budgetary, planning, and goal-setting tools of modern management—to bewail the managerial incompetence of several of the physician department heads. But it is clear that in a head-to-head conflict over the allocation of resources or matters of departmental policy, an MBA is no match for a determined MD. Successful managers are generally those who can skillfully work around the problems caused by the various physician power blocs.

The director of nursing is officially a member of the hospital's senior management group. But much of the nurses' administrative duties concern the patient care unit, or nursing unit. (The term "ward" is never used officially at Parkside, although many older nurses still prefer it to the newer, more abstract term "unit.") Nurses provide the crucial link between the patient and the various clinical and laboratory services that are involved in medical care. Almost all of the hospital's general duty nurses, that is, nonsupervisory RNs who are assigned to a specific medical or surgical unit, carry out some administrative responsibilities in addition to their patient care duties.

Employees and Labor Relations at Parkside

At the time of the quality of work life project, Parkside had over 6000 employees, a figure that has remained relatively constant. Like all modern complex medical centers, Parkside is characterized by a work force that encompasses a vast range of educational and skill levels. For the purposes of this book, it is perhaps best to describe the hospital's employees within the context of the three labor organizations that were formal parties to the quality of work life project and that, in 1975, represented the great majority of Parkside employees. These will be called: the Hospital Workers' Union, which represents technical and non-professional employees; the Parkside chapter of the State Nurses' Association (SNA), which represents all full-time registered nurses who do not have managerial titles at Parkside, and the Parkside Residents' Committee (PRC), which represents the hospital's physicians-in-training or "house staff." The PRC was decertified as a union following the National Labor Relations Board's 1976 ruling that residents and interns are students, not employees, and therefore are not covered by the National Labor Relations Act (see Dworkin, Extejt, & Demming, 1980).

The Hospital Workers' Union. The precursor of the Hospital Workers' Union was organized in the 1930s, but the union did not establish a presence in hospitals until the late 1950s. At that time, the union organized several voluntary hospitals despite the fact that such hospitals were exempt from collective bargaining requirements. Labor relations in the nonprofit hospital sector were chaotic and often strife-torn until the passage of PL 93-360 in 1974, the law that brought (actually, restored) nonprofit hospitals into the framework of the NLRA (Dworkin, Extejt, & Demming, 1980).

The Hospital Workers' Union received considerable support during its formative organizing drives from several prominent civil rights leaders, including Martin Luther King, Jr., A. Philip Randolph, and then-NAACP Counsel Thurgood Marshall. The union maintains close ideological ties to the civil rights movement. During the past twenty years, it has continued to expand its membership; it has organized substantial numbers of professional and technical employees and registered nurses, as well as private nursing home employees. The union's organizing drives aimed at RNs have brought it into substantial conflict with the State Nurses' Association.

The Hospital Workers' Union's impact on wages and fringe benefits has been dramatic. In the late 1950s, prior to unionization, the starting wage of nonprofessional employees at Parkside and comparable voluntary hospitals was as low at $26 a week, and many employees qualified for supplementary public welfare assistance. Fringe benefits were equally meagre; most hospital workers received no hospitalization insurance coverage.

During the 1960s, a decade of low inflation, the wages of hospital workers at Parkside effectively quadrupled as a result of unionization. The union won a guaranteed $100 a week minimum in 1968. Over the years, medical benefits, education and upgrading programs, pensions, and other fringe benefits were added to the contract. By 1976, the first full year of the Parkside Quality of Work Life Project, the average wage of HWU members had reached $228 a week.

HWU's success at the bargaining table has won it the respect and loyalty of its members and the fear of hospital management. The union's successes have also raised the wage expectations of other organized health care groups, including nurses and doctors. Its critics charge that while the HWU is a union that does well by its members economically, it has never been known for its internal democracy. It also has a reputation for going too far in protecting incompetent employees at the expense of patient care. The union's image problem in this area was perhaps one of the factors behind its positive response to the offer to join an experimental joint labor-management program.

At Parkside, the Hospital Workers' Union is headed by two full-time organizers. One represents a division which includes technical, clerical, and professional employees; the other represents the larger division of service and maintenance workers, housekeepers, kitchen employees, and nursing care staff. The organizer of the second division, Moe Kurtzman* was a major figure in the quality of work life project. He and his counterpart in the technical, clerical, and professional division were appointed by the union's citywide leadership. However, organizers come up for re-election every five years.

---

*Again, except where noted, pseudonyms are used throughout the book.

In addition, there is a HWU delegate in each department or major subdivision of Parkside. Delegates are elected every two years. A delegate represents union members in his or her area in the initial stages of the grievance process and usually takes an active role in contract administration. Step three grievances (just before arbitration) are the responsibility of the organizers.

The Parkside Residents' Committee (PRC). In 1975, the Parkside Residents' Committee represented the approximately 350 house staff physicians in the hospital. Residents are medical school graduates who are undergoing a training period of up to eight years in a medical specialization. As part of their training, residents provide almost all of the round-the-clock medical care in the hospital's inpatient units, in the outpatient services, and in the emergency room.

At Parkside as elsewhere, the status of residents is a matter of intense debate. The 1976 NLRB ruling essentially affirmed the position taken by hospital management—that residents are not full professionals with employee status, but rather are students in the final and most demanding phase of medical education. In contrast, PRC's position was that residents are employees and, as licensed physicians, should be accorded greater influence and respect. It charged that residents are overworked, underpaid, and exploited by management under the guise of the "critical learning experience" provided by long, sustained hours on the job and substantial responsibility for patients' lives. Physician administrators of the hospital took the union's charges as evidence of the "soft" attitudes characteristic of a new generation of doctors who are unwilling to accept the demanding regimen faced by previous generations.

Shortly before the start of the quality of work life project, the Parkside Residents' Committee and its counterpart locals in the city's other voluntary and municipal hospitals went on strike over working conditions. The main issues were total work hours per week, the number of consecutive hours on duty, and "out-of-title" work. The union charged that work weeks of 110 hours were not uncommon and that many residents were required to work up to 56 straight hours. The out-of-title complaint alleged that residents were called to perform work that was properly that of nurses and lab technicians. After four days, the strike ended in a settlement that the doctor's union considered a major victory. It limited working hours and set up a joint committee of house staff residents and medical board representatives at each of the hospitals involved to formulate guidelines for work schedules. But the strike also left a residue of bitterness between the union and management. Thus in the following year, in the wake of the NLRB rulings on the status of residents, Parkside management refused to recognize the bargaining status of the Parkside Residents' Committee, a move that effectively destroyed the union. It was no longer a formal part of the quality of work life project.

State Nurses' Association (SNA). The State Nurses' Association is a chapter of the American Nurses' Association. SNA became the collective bargaining representative for registered nurses at Parkside in 1970. At the time of the quality of work life project, the SNA structure in the hospital included a chairman (the term in use), a seven-member executive board, and delegates from each of twelve functional areas within the hospital. In contract matters involving the director of nursing, SNA members are represented by the chairman and the executive board.

Within the hospital, SNA is not looked upon as a particularly militant advocate of its members' interests. Indeed, SNA-affiliated nurses worked without a contract from 1972 until a new contract was finally negotiated in 1974. The question of whether nurses should engage in collective bargaining and pursue trade union interests remains a divisive one within the American Nurses' Association (Aiken, 1983). SNA views itself as an organization dedicated to the professional advancement of nursing and eschews the image of a trade union. Consistent with this position, the 1974 contract in effect at the time of the quality of work life project included substantial funds for professional development and skill upgrading. The contractual grievance process for Parkside nurses calls for the initial discussion of incidents between the nurse and his or her immediate supervisor. If a problem remains, it is referred to the nurse's SNA delegate and to the relevant assistant director of nursing. The third level involves the SNA grievance chairman and the director of nursing. Only rarely does a grievance go beyond the director of nursing to the hospital's director of personnel.

INTERGROUP CONFLICT AT PARKSIDE: A MICROVIEW

Prior to the quality of work life project, doctors, nurses, nonprofessional hospital workers, and hospital administrators had strongly established and generally negative perceptions of one another. The following generalizations are supported by our three years of observational research in the hospital. The day-to-day life on a hospital patient-care unit is dominated by doctors—residents, for the most part—and registered nurses. Conflicts between residents and nurses are readily apparent. Nurses seek full professional recognition; but house staff doctors, who routinely work one hundred or more hours a week, find it difficult to honor the status claims of those who put in a "soft" eight-hour day. Many doctors view nurses as being overly concerned with trivial aspects of the work environment, such as the condition of the locker room or lounge facilities. Residents also view nurses, particularly administrative nurses in charge of nursing floors, as petty bureaucrats or obstructionists who seem concerned with procedures and documentation.

The residents' contact with the hospital workers is much more limited. The tendency among residents is to stereotype nonprofessional class employees and to view them as an undifferentiated mass of workers who carry out their tasks in a perfunctory way and show little concern for the patient care mission. Residents complain about workers who sit around drinking coffee while beds go unmade or bed pans remain unemptied. The typical interaction between a resident and a nursing unit worker is in the form of an order which is often misunderstood and seldom (in the doctor's view) carried out fully. But much of the time, doctors simply ignore hospital workers. Once, in the course of one of our observations of night shift work routines, a resident came into the nursing station looking for a nurse. Two nursing assistants were recording information near the chart rack. There were no nurses about. The doctor called down to a lab department about a particular test and remarked in passing that "there's nobody up here."

Class, race, and gender differences overlay these status and role issues. House staff members are almost exclusively white, and most are males from middle class or upper middle class backgrounds. Male nurses are no longer a rarity; there were four male RNs in general duty and administrative positions on the surgical unit that was the pilot site of the quality of work life project. The ethnic composition of the nursing staff is varied; whites are in the majority but there are significant numbers of Afro-American, Jamaican, Philippino, and Indian nurses. [Nationally, 2 percent of all registered nurses are men; 6 percent of nurses are from minority backgrounds (Moses & Roth, 1978).]. Hospital workers are almost exclusively Hispanic and black, although there are some non-Hispanic white unit clerks. About half of the hospital workers are women.

The nurses' view of intergroup relations is conditioned by an ideology that views patient care as a calling, an ideology that is at the core of the traditional image of the nurse and is reinforced by the work environment of the hospital. But nurses also have come to view themselves as highly skilled professionals who are full participants in the "patient care team." Advances in the technical competence of nursing graduates, particularly, those from baccalaureate nursing programs, add validity to this claim. Aiken, in a recent overview (1983) of the status of nursing, notes that:

> In Nightingale's era, visual observation, touch, sound, and smell were nurses' main assessment tools. Today, nurses monitor the electrical impulses of the heart, measure blood pressure through special lines placed in arteries and veins, assess intracranial pressure by special monitoring devices, examine chests and hearts with stethoscopes, the inner ear with the otoscope, and culture throats, wounds, and urine to determine the presence or absence of bacterial infections. Nurses are also increasingly involved in the direct application of modern medical technologies. They maintain the life support systems of tiny, immature babies in neonatal intensive care units as well as those of comatose adults in the medical-surgical intensive care units. They initiate cardio-pulmonary resuscitation in the event of a cardiac arrest. Specially trained nurses administer anesthesia during surgery, manage renal dialysis units, and deliver babies. [p. 413]

However, in many traditional hospitals, including Parkside, there is a widening gap between what nurses learn in school and what they are allowed to do on the job. Patricia Cayo Sexton, in a recent ethnographic study of hospital workers, succinctly describes the plight of the modern nurse:

> Central to the RN's problems has been nursing's inability to carve out more professional tasks for nurses. Training has been extended and moved out of hospitals and into academics, where it has become more theoretical, less practical and presumably more professional and prestigious; and some routine skills of the RN have been given to others, but few claims to new ground have been staked out. The result for the RN: more years of schooling, an actual shrinking in her scope of practice (on the lower end), and rising frustration at being overschooled for her job. [1982, p. 48]

At Parkside, hospital regulations, traditional interpretations of the physician's role, and autocratic department heads effectively limit claims to professional status by proscribing nurses from carrying out many of the more skilled patient care procedures learned in nursing school. Ironically, overworked residents are usually more than willing to leave such duties as starting IV bottles to the nurses, but hospital rules proscribe this. In turn, nurses are eager to turn over the tedious or unpleasant tasks of patient care to nursing assistants and other nonprofessional staff—in part because of the heavy administrative demands on nurses that intrude upon patient care time, but also because tasks such as cleaning up incontinent patients or changing bed linens hardly mesh with a professional image. The nurses view workers in nonpatient care roles such as messengers, elevator operators, and housekeepers in much the same way that doctors do—as lazy and unconcerned about the mission of the hospital.

Most hospital workers are poorly educated and work outside of any firm professional tradition. Due to the impact of unionization, hospital jobs pay well relative to other forms of unskilled or semiskilled labor and offer a considerably better range of benefits. But hospital workers are fully aware of their position at the bottom of the status hierarchy of the hospital and resent the lack of consideration and respect they receive from other employees.

The Impact of Job Hierarchies

To understand the conflicts between the hospital workers and other employee groups at Parkside, it is important to understand the character of workers' jobs.

Hospital workers carry out tasks which are codified in detailed, formal job descriptions. The worker receives the training necessary to perform his or her particular job and interacts with other types of employees only as job requirements demand. Work conflicts trigger an elaborate set of grievance procedures. When an incident takes place, the union delegate and, if necessary, the union organizer represent the employee to management. The worker is limited to an essentially passive role. The delegate system, which is intended to safeguard employee rights under the contract, can lead to extreme rigidity. Everyday conflicts that common sense suggests should be settled informally between the employee and the supervisor can escalate into major incidents, as illustrated by the following example.

Just before the initiation of the quality of work life project, a dispute arose over who was responsible for cleaning up the feces of incontinent patients. Existing job descriptions gave no explicit attention to the problem nor any indication of whether nurses, nursing aides, or housekeeping personnel should bear the responsibility. Unable to resolve the question, the affected personnel filed a grievance, and the matter was finally settled by arbitration a month later. The arbitrator's decision established strict locational standards. In the bed, cleaning up was the nurse's responsibility; within six inches of the bed, the nursing aide was responsible; beyond six inches of the bed, the task fell to housekeeping personnel. In describing the incident and its aftermath, nurses and nonprofessional workers were fully aware of its ludicrous aspects, but the event illustrates the staff's dependence on mechanisms such as grievance procedures and arbitration to solve problems that could be resolved by informal discussion and negotiation among those involved. Such are a natural outgrowth of a climate of intergroup suspicion, a long tradition of adversarial union-management relations, and the felt need among all parties to provide for all possible exigencies in written contracts. Given the complex, interactive nature of hospital work, however, establishing external standards for everything is clearly impossible.

Consider also the following typical situation: a messenger who carries blood samples from the nursing unit to the laboratory calls in sick on a day when there is no immediate replacement available. The messenger who handles urine samples will not substitute because handling "blood work" is not in his or her job description. When the sample is finally dispatched, it may disappear somewhere in the transfer process between the messenger, the lab clerk, and the technician. After the sample is processed, the record of results may not reach the doctor who ordered the tests. Some doctors deal with the problem by ordering the same test more than once to protect against loss. Not surprisingly, doctors sometimes forget that a specific test was ordered. Down in the laboratory, the technician who had previously tested all types of blood for a variety of diseases may now test only Types O and A for anemia. The reduced job leads to boredom and carelessness, reinforced by the knowledge that ordered tests are often never used. Feedback is seldom given for good performance; more likely, it takes the form of a complaint or reprimand from a supervisor over a lost or inadequately performed task that resulted in a problem for the doctor at the other end of the task chain.

Despite these widely recognized problems, there are important reasons why job fragmentation persists in hospitals and, indeed, may be increasing. Management is concerned with control and efficiency. The simpler a particular task, the easier it is to establish standards for employee evaluation. When the employee fails to perform adequately and must be replaced, job simplification minimizes the training costs of the replacement worker.

On its part, the Hospital Workers' Union favors tightly defined job descriptions. If the job is precisely and contractually specified, employees are protected from having to perform unreasonable tasks. The union seeks to maintain as many different job descriptions as possible—each with a distinct rate of pay. This expands promotion opportunities and increases in pay, however incremental, and allows the union to view itself as a force for employee upgrading. But another result is that the union is often conditioned to resist turning fragmented jobs into more meaningful, challenging ones. Moreover, promotional ceilings in hospitals are relatively low because of the presence of so many licensed occupations. Therefore, expanding the number of new job grades can only result in further job fragmentation.

Apart from these problems, work life within the hospital suffers from basic communications problems among staff members. The typical management approach is to issue directives without communicating the underlying reasons or goals. Moreover, information tends to move in one direction only. Policy is set at the top departmental administrators devise means of implementation, and orders are passed down to functionaries who have been delegated narrowly defined responsibilities. If a lower level employee wants to communicate a message upward, however, it usually stops at the level of his or her immediate supervisor.

The end result can be seen in the story of an employee who suffered a serious off-the-job accident: the man woke up in another hospital, called his supervisor at Parkside, and was told to not worry about returning to work until he was fully recuperated. A few weeks later, his doctor told him that he could return to work on a part-time basis. The employee called the supervisor, who told him to remain at home until he could return to full-time work. Three weeks later, he returned to Parkside ready to assume his regular schedule and was told that he was fired because he had failed to adequately report changes in his condition—in violation of the hospital's policy that disabled employees must return to work on at least a part-time basis as soon as possible. The supervisor had misinformed the employee but did not have the authority to rectify the error. The union filed a grievance which went all the way to arbitration before the employee was finally reinstated. Union officials contend that this is not an unusual case.

Autocratic management thrives in the quasi-military environment of the hospital. Doctors issue orders to nurses, nurses to nursing aides, and aides to orderlies. The order may be valid, but the tone of communication invites passive resistance. The employee "gets back" at the superior by selective intention, by carrying out the order in a literal or perfunctory way, or by refusing the order on the grounds that it violates the job description. The ultimate loser in these exchanges is the patient. Coordinating the myriad functions within the hospital is the purpose of innumerable meetings, but the meetings are usually among peers. Doctors meet with the doctors, unit supervisors meet with other unit supervisors, and so forth. Decisions are made, procedures are adopted, and the outcomes are imposed on lower level staff members who have no direct or representative participation in the process.

Our observation-based impressions of Parkside are highly consonant with other accounts of intergroup relations within contemporary hospitals. We are convinced that, despite the claim that was often made by quality of work life project participants at Parkside—that the hospital was "special" and "more complex" than other medical care settings—many of Parkside's problems are generic to large hospitals. Indeed, many of the features of the hospital that we observed were described over two decades ago by Georgopoulos and Mann in their classic study of the organization of the community general hospital. They note, for example, that

> Work in the hospital is greatly differentiated and specialized, and of a highly interactional character. It is carried out by a large number of cooperating people whose backgrounds, education, training, skills, and functions are as diverse and heterogeneous as can be found in any of the most complex organizations in existence. [1962, p. 100]

Moreover:

> The product of the organization—patient care—is itself individualized rather than uniform or invariant. Because the work is neither mechanized nor uniform or standardized, and because it cannot be planned in advance with the automatic precision of an assembly line, the organization must depend a good deal upon its various members to make the day-to-day adjustments which the situation may demand, but which cannot possibly be completely detailed or prescribed by formal organizational rules and regulations. [p. 100]

At Parkside, such "day-to-day adjustments" are made grudgingly. Weisbord's (1976) comment about hospitals—that "while the systems are extremely interdependent, people do not act that way" (p. 18)—fits Parkside well. This problem leads to what Georgopoulos and Mann call "quasi-authoritarian means of control," such as rigid rules and procedures and close supervision which insure the necessary behavioral compliance. Like most hospitals, Parkside is a mass of contradictions—an arena where employees' need for autonomy in their work makes it necessary to impose bureaucratic order, which frustrates autonomy needs and provokes passive resistance. This in turn leads to more external regulation.

The result of this vicious cycle is an institution that commands respect but little love or organizational commitment among its employees.

Assessing the Potential for Organizational Change at Parkside

Quality of work life programs often begin when a manager or union leader assumes the role of advocate or sponsor for a change effort to improve work relations or organizational performance. This was not the case at Parkside. As described in Chapter 2, the QWL project and the model of organizational change upon which it was based were developed externally as part of a national series of demonstration projects. There were no direct financial costs to the management of the hospital or to the participating unions. The project was "free" also in the sense that it was framed as an experimental effort; there were no commitments to specific outcomes, and individual managers and union leaders were not liable if the project failed. The unusual auspices of the project led to a number of important questions: Who would assume responsibility for the project within the hospital? Where would the energy necessary for a QWL project come from? What would be the impact of the prevailing labor relations climate on the project? And the overriding question: Was Parkside a suitable QWL intervention site?

Clearly, there was a definite need for improving the quality of employee work life at Parkside. Poor communication among staff members at different levels, status insecurity, militant avoidance of "out-of-title" work, and poor scheduling and task coordination characterized the hospital's nursing units. Cynicism and hostility toward the institution permeated employees' break-time conversations. While none of these problems was serious enough to compromise Parkside's first-rank medical reputation, there was common agreement that patient care suffered as a result of Parkside's difficult work environment. One telling example is the advice given by a Parkside senior attending surgeon to a Columbia research team member who was investigating where to have minor surgery performed. The doctor advised "Don't have it done here. Go to a small community hospital in the suburbs somewhere—you'll get better care."

If the need for improving the work climate was evident, it also seemed clear that Parkside's nursing staff would be receptive to the goals of a QWL project. As noted, Parkside RNs were acutely aware of the considerable gap between the level and types of skill acquired in baccalaureate nursing education and the reality of nursing care at Parkside. Nurses were also critically important to every division of the hospital. They formed a large, well-educated constituency for work reform.

But while the need for change at Parkside was apparent to both employees and outside observers, whether or not a joint union-management QWL project was an appropriate vehicle for bringing about such change was another question. In the 1974–75 period, there were several factors that increased the risk of failure of such a project. The most salient problem was the nature of union-management relations at the hospital. Previous research (Nadler, Hanlon, & Lawler, 1980) indicates that the level of trust between labor and management is an important predictor of the success or failure of quality of work life projects. At Parkside, relations between the administration of the hospital and employee groups were marked by extreme mistrust. When the hospital won the legal authority to destroy the house staff union, it acted swiftly in doing so. Pervasive rumors of staff cuts and layoffs undercut attempts to improve communications between the hospital and the Hospital Workers' Union. As we describe later, the incoming director of the hospital at the time the project began believed that a collaborative relationship with the Hospital Workers' Union would be contradictory to the policy of "tighter" management and greater fiscal accountability.

Relations between the unions at Parkside also worked against a successful outcome. The hospital workers were engaged in a chronic dispute with the administration of the department of nursing and had filed several grievances over arbitrary supervisory practices. Since the hospital had no first level supervisory position equivalent to that of unit manager, supervisory authority over HWU members often fell to the most senior registered nurse on duty, who was usually an SNA member. In other hospitals within the metropolitan area, the Hospital Workers' Union was challenging SNA for representation rights for RNs, and it had won a number of elections.

In short, the climate of mistrust that pervaded labor relations in the hospital could be expected to limit the ability of participating groups to practice the kind of integrative bargaining described in Chapter 2.

A second major problem was the size of Parkside Hospital. In a complex 1200 bed facility devoted to patient care, teaching, and research, the site of any successful pilot-type project runs a risk of becoming an "innovation ghetto" (Toch and Grant, 1982)—an encapsulated, highly atypical social unit. As Lawler (1982) points out, organizational change projects must overcome the considerable force of the "principle of congruence": a change that disturbs established organizational patterns is likely to be resisted by any large organization. This is especially likely when the innovation entails radical changes in behavior. The participative, democratic, bottom-up philosophy of QWL is very much at odds with the authoritarian character of work relations in a complex hospital. A successful pilot-level intervention is no guarantee

Table 3.1. Parkside as an Underbounded System

Boundary Parameter	Key Characteristics of Underbounded Systems	Illustrative Characteristics From Parkside
Authority	Nature of authority is unclear; several individuals or groups hold responsibility for the same thing or work not done because no one is assigned to it.	Ambiguity of medical vs. administrative authority, diffuse decision making about patient care, lack of clarity about who makes many decisions.
Role definition	Organizational members uncertain about limits or priorities in their work, resulting in poor planning and response to events on a crisis basis.	Lack of systematic planning of patient care, nursing unit constantly in a state of emergency or crisis because of the lack of planning.
Communication	Problems result when people, kept apart by conflicting demands, do not meet to discuss important issues.	Difficulty of holding meetings either on the nursing unit or the hospital at large because of different schedule and priorities.
Human energy	Difficulties in harnessing energy to do work; people geographically dispersed and pulled in conflicting directions.	People involved in patient care located in different departments and sites with differing time schedules, priorities, etc.
Affect	Expression of affect not constrained but dominantly negative; hostile and anxious feelings expressed towards others and selves.	Frequent and intense expressions of negative feelings by staff on the nursing unit.
Economic condition	Scarcity of funds; relatively great economic uncertainty.	Budget deficit and perception of uncontained costs increase tensions between union and management and reduce willingness to provide staff release time and other resources for innovation.
Time span of concern	Short run; continually facing issues of survival; crisis-oriented mentality.	Emphasis on dealing with immediate crises, not longer-range strategies for work and organizational reform.

Source. Adapted from Nadler (1978).

that the project can be expanded to larger organizations or that innovations will last. The question of the institutionalization of change is one of the most difficult challenges facing QWL advocates and one that has generated a great deal of recent attention (Goodman, 1979; Goodman & Dean, 1982). It is a theme that we will consider in the concluding chapter of this book.

A third problem is related to the organizational structure of the hospital. Typical of most hospitals, Parkside has many of the characteristics of what Alderfer (1976) terms an "underbounded system." The boundaries between organizational units are easily permeable and often poorly defined. Nowhere is this more clear than in a typical nursing care unit. At Parkside, the staff assigned to a nursing unit number about 25, but high turnover rates, particularly among RNs, and the floating of staff persons to other units during peak demand periods work against the formation of stable work groups. Attending physicians, who use the resources of the nursing unit and who often place difficult demands on its staff, have no formal ties to the unit and its work system. Patients live in the nursing unit throughout their stay, but much of their medical treatment is rendered elsewhere in the hospital. The inability of unit staff to maintain cohesive boundaries and thus a sense of control over the work process is at the heart of many complaints about the quality of work life in the unit. This problem is expressed clearly in the comment of a senior nurse of one of the hospital's surgical nursing units:

> Sometimes I come back from lunch, and it feels like chaos. I don't know where my patients are, half the charts are out of the rack, and the blood bank is on the phone, angry. That's when you feel like giving up—like just walking away from the place.

Table 3.1 summarizes the problematic features of the hospital structure at the time of the initiation of the quality of work life project. These characteristics are based on Alderfer's (1976) discussion of underbounded systems and on our diagnostic research at Parkside.

In summary, Parkside Hospital at the time of the QWL project was an institution where the need to improve working life and to increase operating effectiveness was very evident. It was an open question, however, whether the necessary solutions would be able to overcome the problematic nature of labor relations, the size of the institution, and the peculiar structural characteristics of the hospital.

HISTORY OF THE PARKSIDE QUALITY OF WORK LIFE PROJECT

INTRODUCTION

In the five chapters that follow, we present a detailed history of the Parkside Quality of Work Life Project. Our main objective is to provide a sense of the complexity of this type of organizational intervention within the context of a tertiary care hospital affiliated with a major medical school. We attempt to convey the flavor of the project while providing our interpretation of its progress. As much as possible, we trace the course of the project from the perspective of the team of consultants that was hired to facilitate change and provide technical expertise to the principal policy-making body of the project—the joint union-management steering committee. We follow the consultants as they try to make sense of a diffuse and complex system, a novel type of client (a joint union-management committee), and an extremely challenging task—making the hospital more effective in providing high quality patient care by increasing employee participation in decision making.

The Parkside QWL Project did not follow a simple and consistent course. Much of what happened was, of course, idiosyncratic to Parkside. But we also believe that many of the types of problems encountered by the consultants and project participants are generic to large, modern-day medical care organizations. As much as possible, we have tried to keep these general points in mind throughout the course of this detailed case study.

The narrative follows the five major stages of the Parkside Quality of Work Life Project and covers a range of events beginning from the October 1973 meeting with the president of the union that represented the largest group of employees in the hospital through the Columbia

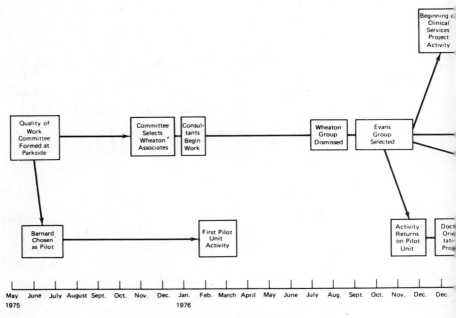

Figure 1. Parkside QWL project:

research team's final assessment interviews in February of 1979. The major events in the history of the project are summarized in chronological form (Table 1) and diagramatically (Figure 1).

This history is based largely on our three years of observation at Parkside and on interviews with participants in the project.

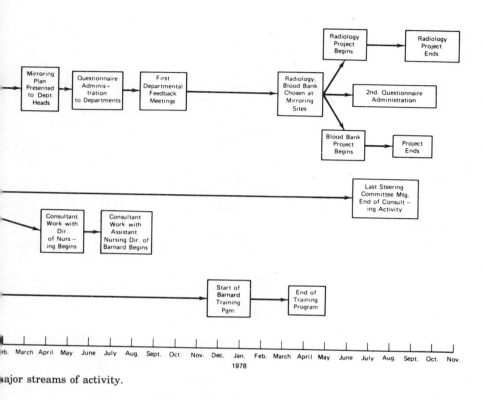

... ajor streams of activity.

Table 1. Parkside Quality of Work Life Project: Significant Events

Date	Event
1974	
July	Parkside management approves Project.
1975	
March	Joint meeting of HWU, State Nurses' Association, Parkside Residents' Committee.
May	First joint union-management meeting (5/7). Union management committee (later called the Project Steering Committee) is set up.
Preproject Period	
1973	
October	First discussions between National Quality of Work Life Center and Hospital Workers' Union (HWU).

45

Table 1. *(Continued)*

Date	Event
Preproject Period	
1975	
May	Union-management committee selects a surgical nursing unit, Barnard 5, as the initial project pilot site (5/21).
September	First QWL Project staff meeting on Barnard 5 (9/29).
December	Wheaton Associates team selected as project consultants (12/5).
The Project Begins:	
The Wheaton Associates Period	
1976	
January	Project Steering Committee and Barnard 5 Task Force hold first working meeting with Wheaton team (1/9).
	Wheaton consultant team's first meeting on Barnard 5 (1/22).
February	First HEW site visit (2/27). Project receives favorable review.
February (through June)	Period of increased tension between HWU and hospital management. First layoff threats.
May	NQWC, Columbia research team and steering committee hold emergency meeting to discuss problems with the Wheaton intervention.
June	Ten-day Hospital Workers' Union strike against several area voluntary hospitals including Parkside.
August	Wheaton Associates team terminated as project consultants (8/6).
A New Beginning	
The Early Stages of the Evans Consultation	
September	Evans' team selected as project consultants (9/8).
October	Evans presents initial QWL Project Organization Development Plan to the steering committee (10/12).
1977	
January	Staff conferences begin on Barnard 5. Barnard 5 staff hold first orientation for new surgical residents.
	Evans holds first meeting with Assistant Director of Barnard Pavilion, Nancy Marullo, to define her role in QWL Project.
	The Evans team presents briefing on Project to the Parkside Senior Management Group (1/24).
February	The Evans team fails to win support for its proposal to restructure the steering committee.

Table 1. *(Continued)*

Date	Event
March	Scheduling crisis on Barnard 5 jeopardizes project gains. Consultants vow to seek high level management support (3/7).

Building Ownership:
The Evolution of the Consultants' Strategy

Date	Event
March	Consultants hold meetings with Hospital Workers' Union leadership in the hospital to build union involvement. Evans proposes an HWU training program.
April	Evans begins consulting work with Director of Nursing Meredith Klein.
May	Hartman and the director of clinical services present survey feedback project plan to clinical services department directors (5/11). Administration of the first survey feedback questionnaire. Moe Kurtzman of HWU returns to the steering committee.
June	Evans begins intensive consulting work with Nancy Marullo, Assistant Director of Nursing for Barnard Pavilion, and her staff. Evans' team presents briefing on QWL Project status to the steering committee (6/7). Midpoint of the Evans' consulting contract.
October	Consultants' steering committee restructuring plan is approved (10/7). An executive working group is formed. Full steering committee will not meet again until the end of the project.

Maturation and Decline:
The Second Half of the Evans Consultation

Date	Event
December	First training program session. Program continues through March of 1978.
1978	
March	Radiology and blood bank chosen as pilot sites for the organization mirroring project.
April	Blood bank/nursing mirroring group begins a series of meetings that continue through July. Radiology/nursing mirroring group begins a series of meetings that continue through December.
June	Final steering committee meeting (6/6). Evans presents recommendations for diffusion of project activities.
July	Second clinical services survey feedback project questionnaire. Poor response rate. Most departments do not intend to use the data.
August	Official project termination date (8/31).

CHAPTER FOUR

The Origins of the Parkside Quality of Work Life Project

In October of 1973, a representative of the National Quality of Work Center (NQWC), the organization that was responsible for initiating the different projects within the Michigan Quality of Work Program, met with the president of the Hospital Workers' Union to discuss the possibility of a quality of work life demonstration project in a large urban hospital. The Hospital Workers' Union was approached because of its prominent role within the health care sector in the eastern United States. The NQWC representative explained to the union president that should HWU decide to participate in a demonstration project, the union would have the right to choose the specific site—presumably, a hospital or health care facility where union-management relations were secure enough to allow for collaborative activity. As a matter of strategy, it was important that the union side be dealt with before management entered the picture. At this point in the evolution of the quality of work life movement, most major unions were wary of collaborative projects, particularly where improvements in productivity or service capability created a fear of layoffs or uncompensated "speed-ups." Allowing the union to select the site reduced suspicion of the project.

The leadership of HWU was convinced that the project offered the promise of significant benefits for workers. The project also provided a means of publicly affirming the union's commitment to quality patient care. The union selected Parkside Hospital as the tentative project site—largely because the hospital's vice president for personnel was a prominent figure in the health care labor relations field. HWU viewed him as tough but fair; he also had the advantage of being a known quantity.

MAKING CONTACT WITH PARKSIDE MANGEMENT

With HWU's approval, a representative from NQWC contacted Parkside's vice president for personnel, who was receptive immediately to the idea of a participative effort with the union. Discussions between the NQWC's representative and the vice president for personnel and his staff led to a consensus over the general location of the project; it should be in an area of the hospital devoted to direct patient care rather than to clerical or "hotel service" functions. Also, since patient care involved complex interactions between different types of employees, it was essential to bring in the two other major employee groups at Parkside: the State Nurses' Association and the Parkside Residents' Committee. Patient participation or representation was also suggested but due to the transience of patients, the group felt that this should be dealt with at a later stage once the project was solidly established.

Subsequent meetings were held with the hospital's newly appointed director, Harvey Hertz, and ten other senior managers. All expressed approval, and some were genuinely enthusiastic.

CONTACTS WITH THE STATE NURSES' ASSOCIATION

The NQWC representative then met with the state president and regional director of the State Nurses' Association and later with the five nurses who comprised the executive committee of the SNA chapter at Parkside. If anything, the nurses' group was even more enthusiastic than HWU or Parkside management about the idea of a collaborative project. As described in Chapter 3, nurses viewed their role in the hospital as pivotal but problematic. Conflict, particularly between physicians and nurses, severely limited the nurses' effectiveness and stifled their claims to full professional status. A quality of work life project would provide a potentially useful vehicle for dealing with these sensitive issues.

APPROACHING THE PARKSIDE RESIDENTS' COMMITTEE

The NQWC representative contacted the Parkside Residents' Committee through the attorney who represented PRC in contract negotiations. He was cooperative and indicated that he would recommend participation to the PRC leadership. However, he was skeptical about the prospect of any collaborative relationship with the management of the hospital. He stated that as a negotiator who had been engaged in almost constant battles with management over the past three years (a period in which PRC had won substantial gains in pay and fringe benefits), he felt confident that management would be unwilling to give up any real control in the context of a QWL project and would seek to use the project to extract gains they would not otherwise win.

In fact, follow-up meetings with PRC leadership revealed a great deal more interest in the project than the attorney had expected. In early 1975, PRC held a strike at Parkside Hospital. PRC (and its counterparts in other voluntary hospitals in the city) won some of its demands but the experience left it exhausted and more receptive to an opportunity to deal with management on a nonadversarial basis. PRC found itself pleasantly surprised that Parkside management had agreed to participate in a collaborative project with several unions. In addition, the doctors felt that such a project would provide a means of reviewing the numerous hospital procedures and rules that caused friction between house staff and other groups involved in patient care. As noted in Chapter 3, many of the young physicians at Parkside were more than willing to turn over responsibility for many patient care procedures to RNs, who in turn were seeking to expand their own skills and prerogatives. From PRC's perspective, discovering such complementary interests and helping to bring about mutually beneficial changes would be among the important functions of a collaborative intergroup project.

THE FIRST JOINT UNION MEETING

In early March of 1975, eight months after Parkside management had given its approval for the project, the leadership of the three unions— the Hospital Workers' Union, the State Nurses' Association, and the Parkside Residents' Committee—met with National Quality of Work Center staff members at a luncheon meeting at the Hospital Workers' Union headquarters. To the best of participants' knowledge, it was the first time that all three unions had come together for any purpose.

The NQWC staff started the meeting by offering a summary statement on the objectives of a quality of work life project—even though all three employee groups were familiar with QWL by this time. It was important to get across the point that all three unions were equal participants and privy to the same information. Then the discussion was thrown open for suggestions and reactions.

The regional president of HWU reaffirmed the union's belief that a major goal of the project should be to make the membership more aware of the basic purpose of the hospital: to provide quality patient care. His statement found widespread support; the theme of the ensuing discussion was how easy it was to lose sight of patient well-being amid the pressing demands of hospital work.

The SNA representatives took a different position. They asserted that management often used the ideal of patient care to justify additional, often unreasonable demands on hospital personnel. For the project to work, management would have to commit itself to a sincere joint effort and forego the temptation to use quality of working life as a means of getting more work out of already overextended employees. That being said, SNA joined in the general celebration of the uniqueness of the event and the potential gains to be had from the project.

The group turned next to the choice of the specific locale within the hospital that would serve as the project site. At this point, the NQWC representatives pointed out that only labor was represented at this meeting; the choice of the project site should wait until the first joint union-management meeting. The group fully agreed. Tabling site selection until the first joint meeting reinforced the sense among the union representatives that they were embarking on a truly collaborative venture where both sides would have an equal voice.

THE FIRST JOINT UNION-MANAGEMENT MEETINGS

On May 7, 1975 (some eighteen months after the first contacts with the Hospital Workers' Union), representatives of the three unions, Parkside management, the National Quality of Work Center, and the Institute for Social Research of the University of Michigan came together to launch the Parkside Quality of Work Life Project. A QWL Committee was set up, the structure of which is presented in Figure 4.1.

Like the earlier joint union meeting, the first order of business was a statement by the NQWC representative about the general objectives and scope of the project. Again, the purpose was less an informational one than a matter of establishing the norm that all constituent groups should have an equal say. At the NQWC representative's suggestion, the group went directly to the key issue of site selection. Most of the management representatives present, including the outgoing director of the hospital, favored a specific department such as radiology or a hospital service function such as transport and information. This was a definite change from the early opinion of the vice president for personnel that a patient care unit should be the focus of the project. (The vice president for personnel did not attend the first joint union-management meeting, and his role was extremely limited throughout the subsequent history of the project.) The management representatives said that it would be much easier to measure project results in a functional area than in a diffuse patient care unit. Also, a previous effort to increase employee participation on a patient care unit had been tried and had failed.

These were the manifest reasons for management's change of heart. But the Columbia research team also sensed that management felt a growing fear that a project that was cosponsored by the unions could "get out of hand." In defensive terms, a project in a functional area such as transport and information could be controlled by the existing management hierarchy; on a nursing floor, line management authority was relatively weak.

All three unions strongly opposed management's point of view. Representatives argued that a functional department such as "T&I" provided limited direct contact between patients, doctors, nurses, and hospital workers. A clinical department—radiology, for example—involved direct patient contact but in a highly specialized context. In either of these situations, the uniqueness of the site would hinder duplication of successful outcomes. From a research perspective (here the three Parkside Residents' Committee representatives took the initiative), the selection of a unique department would make it impossible to come up with a suitable control site within the hospital. Finally, the earlier nursing unit failure cited by management was hardly a precedent; the QWL project had the support of all major constituent groups—it could not be dismissed as a management gimmick, and it deserved the support of hospital employees. Also, as the NQWC representative had noted in his early contacts with the unions and with management, the project, if it was approved and funded, would have the services of a behavioral science-trained consultant team that would provide participants with the various skills necessary for a successful project.

With one voice, the unions argued that a nursing unit should be the site of the project. Patients on a nursing unit receive virtually every service provided by the hospital, and all hospital employees who have direct patient contact, from senior physicians to nursing aides, interact on the nursing unit. With the exception of resident physicians, who rotate between medical services every two to six months, the staff on a nursing unit is relatively stable. A unit is a complex, twenty-four hour operation, and each of the three shifts involves a different mix of patient care responsibilities. Also, the hospital had over thirty nursing units—many of them roughly comparable in functions and staffing configurations—so that project outcomes, good or bad, would offer lessons applicable elsewhere. The similarities among units would also allow for control or comparison sites. Finally, the unions argued that communication problems seemed to underly most of the conflicts between staff members, and the nursing unit would offer the most important sites for improving communications.

Faced with these arguments, management backed down; by consensus, the group decided to select a nursing unit as the initial project site.

Choosing a specific unit was not easy. Several units were mentioned as possible sites, but the decision could not be imposed on unit level employees. That would be contrary to the participative ethos of the project, and it probably wouldn't work. The union-management group decided to form an ad hoc working group consisting of one representative from each of the unions and one from management. The small group would spend a couple of weeks assessing employee attitudes on different nursing units and then select the most favorable site.

Up to this point, the actual composition of the permanent union-management body was given little explicit consideration. Now, the NQWC representative urged the group to consider its official structure. Several alternative forms were considered in the subsequent discussion, ranging from a high level committee made up of key representatives from different areas of the hospital to a multilevel group that would include several employees from the designated nursing unit. Ultimately, the group decided to form a basically unit level committee, but one that would include one non-unit management representative, one nursing supervisor (considered as management), two HWU representatives (including the union delegate on the unit), two staff nurses, two PRC-affiliated resident physicians, and a unit-based HWU-affiliated social worker. The composition of the group was tentative at this point since the actual pilot unit had not been selected and there was no assurance that unit staff would accept the proposed system of representation. The meeting ended with some discussion of the future of the larger union-management group—specifically, the details of when it would meet again, how often it would meet, and whether it would be a permanent component of the project. None of these questions produced a clear answer.

The second joint union-management meeting took place on May 21, 1975. It was arranged as a meeting of the small ad hoc committee that was charged with selecting a pilot unit. However, several additional people, all of whom were affiliated with hospital management, came to the meeting. Because of this influx of new members, the group was forced to go back over much of the same introductory ground covered in the first meeting. The group was unsure of its boundaries and functions and could not decide if this was a meeting of the ad hoc site selection committee or a somewhat reduced version of the full union-management group.

Again, the NQWC representative took an active leadership role. In the two weeks since the first meeting he had been sounding out officials in different areas of the hospital in order to come up with possible project sites. The chief of medicine wanted the pilot project on a unit within his jurisdiction, but the NQWC representative uncovered substantial resistance to the project among nursing staff within the division of medicine. The ad hoc committee then considered a psychiatric unit and a private care unit but eventually rejected both; the former was too idiosyncratic and the latter, with thirty or so attending physicians, was too complicated. Other suggested sites were quickly ruled out for a variety of practical reasons.

Then Blanche Reiner, an assistant director of social service who was an active participant in the early meetings, described an employee participation experiment on Barnard 6, a unit in one of the hospital's older surgical pavilions. The experiment was being carried out by the department of community medicine. It was not a joint union-management effort but, Reiner noted, it would offer an interesting comparison site. The group quickly agreed to her suggestion that Barnard 5, the unit immediately below community medicine's experimental unit, should be approached to become the pilot site of the QWL project.

Defining the Parkside Steering Committee

By selecting a tentative site for the project, the union-management group had completed its first task successfully. Still, the group lacked certain essential elements that seriously compromised its effectiveness. These were: a name, a long-term mandate, and defined boundaries. Throughout this early period, the group relied heavily on the NQWC representative for leadership; it was not an independent, self-sustaining working group. Nor did it have a clearly defined membership, although during these early meetings, a leadership group emerged that remained throughout the life of the project. The group included:

Moe Kurtzman. The full-time union organizer for the 2000 non-professional class Hospital Workers' Union members in the hospital. By virtue of his position and dynamic personal style, Kurtzman was a dominant figure in the early stages of the project.

Blanche Reiner. The Assistant Director of Social Services at Parkside. Reiner was the chief administrator for in-patient social work programs in the hospital and an instructor in the department of community medicine in the medicine school. Reiner's participation in the quality of work life project was motivated by her interest in expanding employee involvement in the delivery of health care.

Meredith Klein. Parkside's Director of Nursing. Klein assumed the position a year before the start of the QWL project. She was the first director of nursing to sit on the hospital's executive body, the Parkside Senior Management Group. She viewed herself as a member of management, not as an advocate of nurses as an interest group in the hospital.

Dr. Arthur Saltzman. Surgeon and Associate Professor of Surgery at Parkside Medical School. Saltzman, the one physician at Parkside who took an early and sustained interest in the QWL project, provided strong, task-oriented leadership within the union-management group. Saltzman had absolutely no previous experience in behavioral science-based organizational change projects, but he saw the quality of work life project as a means of reducing the irrational boundaries that separated different types of employees and reduced the quality of patient care.

Sally McBride. McBride joined the group as the representative of the State Nurses' Association, despite the fact that she had been defeated recently for reelection as chairman of the SNA local chapter. She had limited personal influence within the union-management group.

Loretta Musial. Director of Training and Development at Parkside. Musial reported to the vice president for personnel. She was responsible for all "housekeeping" functions related to the QWL project including the production and distribution of minutes, scheduling lunches, and so on.

The third meeting of the group, which took place on June 17, was devoted largely to important issues of role and structure. David Nadler of the Columbia research team took an active role in defining the separate functions of the union-management committee and of the eventual working group on Barnard 5, the nursing unit selected as the pilot unit for the project. Nadler's proposals were consistent with the ISR Quality of Work Model described in Chapter 2. By the end of the meeting, participants had agreed on the following:

The hospital-level union-management group would be called the Project Steering Committee. It would be the hospital's executive policy-making body of the quality of work life project, and its specific functions would include:

1.   Overall management of the various QWL activities at Parkside
2.   Serving as the primary contact for outside groups, including the consultant team, funding agencies, the National Quality of Work Center, and the Columbia research team
3.   Review and oversight responsibility for specific projects
4.   Serving as the basic forum for the exchange of ideas between unions and management on improving quality of work life
5.   Serving as a neutral party in any intergroup conflicts that might arise in the course of the project

Nadler described the role of the steering committee as the "hub of the wheel." The group would coordinate the activities of each of the unit, service, or department level task forces, beginning with the group on Barnard 5. In turn, each of the task forces or working groups would have its own sphere of responsibility that would include:

1.   Working with the consultant team in diagnosing problems and planning change strategies
2.   Working with the Columbia research team in collecting information about the effectiveness or impact of project-related changes
3.   Representing the different employee groups on the unit, service, or department level
4.   Providing regular status reports to the steering committee

By taking an active role in proposing a specific structure for the QWL project at Parkside, Nadler was clearly going beyond the role of disinterested researcher and evaluator. But the research team felt that outside intervention was necessary at this critical early stage because of the newness of the quality of work concept and the seeming inability of the labor-management group to translate goodwill and enthusiasm into an effective structure for carrying out the goals of the project. The weak boundaries of the group, indicated by the difficulty faced in establishing rules of membership, were especially worrisome to the research team. At each meeting, the number of participants who directly or indirectly represented the interests of management continued to grow.

There were other reasons for concern. Moe Kurtzman, the representative of the Hospital Workers' Union, argued that the freedom of action of project task forces should be limited—a position that was premature in the extreme as the Barnard 5 Task Force had not even been formed at this point. The steering committee was becoming increasingly hostile toward the NQWC representative. Committee members saw him as too directive and unwilling to give up the leadership role, but they were also acutely aware of how much they still depended on him for guidance. With these issues in mind, Nadler suggested to the group that a process consultant be brought in to work with the group to make it more effective in its early stages of development. The steering committee agreed to the suggestion. The process consultant attended almost all of the committee's meetings over the next several months and made some progress in helping the group to overcome its early identity crisis.

Selecting a QWL Consultant Team

By the fourth meeting of the steering committee, which took place on July 1, 1975, the group had received word that the Health Services Administration of the U.S. Department of Health, Education & Welfare had made a firm commitment to fund the project. This meant that the steering committee now faced the task of selecting a consultant—actually, a consultant team, since the scale of the project would demand more than what a single behavioral science consultant could provide. But at this point, the steering committee had little confidence in its ability to make an informed choice, since it had little sense of what the consultant team would actually do. The group turned to Nadler for clarification; he and the NQWC representative outlined the role of the consultant and pointed out that the criteria for selection must be established by the steering committee and not by the outside group.

By the end of the meeting, the steering committee had developed specific criteria for an acceptable consulting team: it must have previous experience in a large hospital setting (many steering committee members emphasized the enormous complexity of the hospital and its uniquely important mission—the preservation of human life); it must have experience in urban settings; and it must have special competence in dealing with issues of ethnicity. Then the steering committee turned to the question of how much input the employee task force on the pilot nursing unit, Barnard 5, should have in the selection of the consultant. After much debate, the steering committee decided that its own role would be to (1) screen the résumés of consultant applicants, (2) prepare a short list of suitable consultant groups, (3) interview these groups, and (4) select the two or three most qualified consultant groups. The final consultant choice would be left in the hands of the Barnard 5 Task Force.

For two months, starting in early September of 1975, the steering committee met every week, and in retrospect, it was the busiest and most exhilarating period in the group's three-year history. First, the committee reviewed the written materials submitted by the thirteen consultant groups that had been solicited by the prime contractor for the project, the Institute for Social Research of the University of Michigan or by David Nadler of the Columbia research team. The committee winnowed the pool down to six groups; factors such as lack of hospital experience, incomplete sets of background materials (missing curriculum vitae, references and so forth), and late applications were used as criteria in rejecting groups. Four of the six groups were interviewed subsequently by the full steering committee. The committee prepared an exercise to test the competence of each consultant group. Early in the interview, the group was given a description of Barnard 5 which included a litany of the unit's problems, including low staff morale, high turnover, and rigid job descriptions. In the interview, the consultants would first read the case description and then answer a series of predetermined questions put to them by different members of the steering committee. These included questions on how the consultants would address these problems in their intervention plan, what the consultants expected of different members of the steering committee, and how patients could be brought into the process of changing the often depressing atmosphere on the nursing floor. The formal, almost ritualized interviewing procedure brought a large measure of fairness to the process insofar as each of the groups was asked the same questions in precisely the same order. But the real function of this procedure was to reduce the anxiety of members of the steering committee. Asking prearranged questions helped to obscure the group's basic quandary: It had little sense of what kind of consultant team it wanted or needed.

The committee dutifully followed its formal script in each of the four interviews. One consultant team was written off almost immediately because of what the steering committee felt was a nervous and ill-prepared presentation. The three remaining teams were given serious attention, but each had manifest limitations as well as strengths.

The first team, Hammond Associates, consisted of four consultants, including a woman and a black. The team leader was a white male physician. The team had considerable health care experience and because of its background and composition, it was given serious attention by the steering committee. The Hammond consultants emphasized interpersonal rather than technical solutions in their answers to the committee's questions. Ironically, the team's performance was characterized by extremely poor interpersonal process; the head consultant was domineering and frequently interrupted the other three. However, this did not affect the steering committee's highly favorable impression of the group.

The other two consultant groups were made up of white males exclusively. The second group to be interviewed was headed by Bill Evans and included two other consultants, Steve Meyer and Dan Hartman. Like Hammond Associates, the Evans team stressed the need for interpersonal solution to problems. The consultants seemed to work well together, and the steering committee was favorably impressed by the group's presentation. After the meeting, however, Dr. Saltzman, the surgeon and medical school professor who had been recruited for the steering committee, asserted that the group had little health care experience. This wasn't true; indeed, the Evans team had made several references to previous work in hospitals and other health care settings. Perhaps because of Saltzman's status as a high ranking physician in the hospital, no one challenged his assertion.

The third and final group was from Wheaton Associates, a large multioffice management consulting firm that was best known for designing employee compensation plans. The team consisted of four white male consultants: Eric Moore, Carl Goode, Art Dowling, and Mirv Weinglass. Their presentation style was much more in the mainstream of traditional management consulting than the informal, interpersonal approach of the other two groups. In his opening remarks, Moore described his consulting method as one of "finding out what people should be doing and figuring out how to get them to do it." Members of the steering committee disliked Moore, and as the meeting continued and the intensity of their feeling became more obvious, Art Dowling began to take control of the consultant team's responses. After the meeting, steering committee members made several favorable comments about Dowling and Goode and expressed concern that Moore would be on the team. (Weinglass said almost nothing during the meeting and aroused no opinions.) Indeed, Blanche Reiner asked if the steering committee could request that Moore be excluded from the Wheaton team if it was chosen for the consultant role. Edward Lawler of the University of Michigan, the principal investigator of the QWL Program of which Parkside was part, answered that the steering committee was the client and that it could negotiate the terms it wanted.

The steering committee ended its part of the consultant selection process with no clear first choice but with three groups that it could live with. At this point, several committee members expressed reservations about turning over the final decision to the staff on Barnard 5. Their arguments were reasonable enough: The unit task force did not exist as a formally organized group (the NQWC representative had been directed to get the group together, but he had not done so yet), and no one knew if Barnard 5 staff had any interest in being the centerpiece of the quality of work life project. There was a time factor. The steering committee met sixteen times between the initial union-management meeting in May and the selection of the three finalists for the consultant position in late October. If it took another six months to form the Barnard 5 Task Force and make the final consultant decision, much of the energy would be drained from the project. The steering committee was impatient with the slow pace and wanted to see some results.

There was still another dimension. The steering committee had worked very intensively over these months and had forged itself into a trusting, if not very efficient, working group. It felt a strong sense of ownership for the project. When the NQWC representative and the process consultant first pointed out the committee's misgiving about the unit task force might be related to reluctance to transfer control, committee members strongly rejected this suggestion. But after heated debate, Blanche Reiner summed up the committee's new realization: "I hear what these guys are telling us. How do we let go of this project; how do we bow out?"

After considerable soul searching the committee decided that it would still have an important role after the focus of attention shifted to Barnard 5. The "hub of the wheel" metaphor seemed to fit, although no one was sure of how often the group would meet or what it would actually do. The immediate task at hand was to decide the number of choices to be given to the Barnard 5 Task Force. Dr. Saltzman, who had quickly assumed a leadership role in the steering committee, summarized its options: It could send the task force the application materials of all three consultant groups, it could eliminate Wheaton and send the task force materials on the other two groups, or it could simply inform the unit group that it had made a choice and ask for ratification. The process consultant then suggested that the task force should be given time to meet; if it showed itself to be a capable group, then the steering committee might feel more comfortable with its original decision to send the task force material on all three consultant groups. The committee agreed. It decided to dispatch four representatives—Kurtzman, Saltzman, and two nursing department representatives from Barnard Pavilion—to meet with the Barnard 5 Task Force.

There were two meetings between the steering committee representatives and staff members on Barnard 5 at the end of October and the beginning of November of 1975. The first meeting was an overall briefing on the project. The second meeting was devoted to the ground rules of consultant choice. At this meeting Bruce Gould, a Barnard 5 RN who had assumed the role of task force leader, first suggested that the steering committee should make an informed choice. His colleagues agreed. But as the discussion continued, the unit group's preference shifted: It wanted to have a hand in selecting the consultants. At the end of the meeting Gould turned to the NQWC representative and said:

> If you say that all three groups are competent, then the important thing is how we feel about them—what vibrations we get from them. Therefore, we have to interview them.

The meeting had a noticeable effect on the steering committee representatives. Afterwards Dr. Saltzman remarked that the task force had shown a real commitment to the project and that the steering committee's only remaining choice was whether to send the unit group information on all three consultant groups or on just two. By this time, it was learned that Eric Moore would be the principal on-site consultant for the Wheaton group—a fact that greatly disturbed the steering committee. But the committee was confident that if the performance of the consultant groups in the second round of interviews was similar to the first round, then the Wheaton group would be out of the running. The third choice would be little more than symbolic. Blanche Reiner's informal tally of preferences within the steering committee revealed that the Evans group and the Hammond team were dead even. No one supported Wheaton. There did not seem to be any reason to assume that the Barnard 5 Task Force would take a radically different position.

The task force interviewed the three consultant teams in separate meetings in November and early December. By the time the interviews were completed it was clear that Gould's initial position was a correct one: The decision should have been left to the steering committee. The Barnard 5 staff had almost no idea of what the project was about. They relied very heavily on the NQWC representative for direction. Moreover, the term task force implied a formal entity that was hardly evident to an outside observer. About half a dozen staff members, including one or two residents, attended each of the the consultant interview meetings but only two members—Bruce Gould and another RN—attended all three. Among the staff members who attended the meetings with the Evans and Hammond teams, the choice was for Evans. Among those who attended the meetings with Hammond and Wheaton, the choice was for Wheaton. Staff members disliked the overbearing style of the leader of the Hammond group. They liked the informality and flexibility of the Evans group but felt that the Wheaton consultants were more knowledgeable—they seemed like "experts."

On December 5, 1975, the unit task force met for the sixth time and, by a split vote, selected the team from Wheaton Associates as project consultants. The half dozen staff members present seemed very anxious about their decision. They asked the NQWC representative if it was irreversible. He replied that it was not; if things didn't work out, the group would have the opportunity to make a change. This seemed to reduce the group's uncertainty about the consequences of their decision.

INTERPRETIVE SUMMARY

The consultant selection phase ended on an unexpected and ironic note in the choice of a team that had no support within the union-management steering committee. Worse, the newly designated on-site consultant was the least liked member of the team. The most ironic twist of all was that the deciding task force vote was cast by the unit social worker who was not even present when the Wheaton team was interviewed.

The decision overshadowed the considerable accomplishments of the pre-start-up phase of the project. These included:

1.   The formation of a unique, union-management working group within an essentially hostile labor relations climate, a group that recognized that all parties had legitimate interests in improving the quality of work life and that existing labor-management structures and processes were not suitable for serving these interests.

2.   The selection of a project site. The negotiations between the unions and management indicated considerable willingness to compromise and to work through opposing interests. The fact that the union

position prevailed in the selection of a nursing unit over a functional area or clinical department symbolized that this would not be a management-dominated project in which labor would be reduced to an advisory role.

3. The structure of the two principal entities of the project—the union-management steering committee and the site level task forces—were defined. This task had required considerable outside input, however.

4. The steering committee carried out its first major task, the selection of the consultant finalists. Members seemed more interested in testing the character of the consultants than in learning from them or getting an idea of what it would be like to work with each of the groups. But the group produced a rational set of criteria for evaluating the consultants and, but for the last-minute decision to include the Wheaton team among the finalists, it was a remarkably successful first attempt at joint union-management problem solving.

But in the end, the steering committee was left with a group it didn't want. The fledgling Barnard 5 Task Force felt the uneasiness of having made a poor and basically uninformed choice—one that would have consequences far beyond the boundaries of the nursing unit. Having no established criteria for selecting the consultant, their decision was based on what seemed to matter in the hospital: the impression of authority. Dressed in conservative three-piece business suits and speaking the jargon of management consulting ("bottom line," "work flow analysis," "results-oriented") the Wheaton team was both incomprehensible and overwhelming. In hindsight, the consultant choice issue underscores the need for educating all key participants about the nature of what quality of work life improvement efforts involve *before* important decisions are made. But at the time, this was obvious to no one, including the social scientists who designed, sponsored, and evaluated the Parkside project.

CHAPTER FIVE

The Project Begins
The Wheaton Associates Period

With the long consultant selection process over, the action phase of the Parkside Quality of Work Life Project was finally underway. January 9, 1976 was the date set for the Wheaton consulting team to meet with their clients, the Parkside Steering Committee and the Barnard 5 Task Force. An outsider viewing the project for the first time might have wondered about its nature from the participants at the meeting. Seated around a large oval conference table in the ornate boardroom of one of the hospital's older buildings were the four Wheaton consultants, the four-member Columbia research group, and the representative from the National Quality of Work Center. In contrast, only three members of the Parkside Steering Committee were present (Gertrude Thayer, Sally McBride, and Moe Kurtzman) along with two representatives of the Barnard 5 Task Force (Bruce Gould and Nancy Baldwin). Ms. Baldwin, who had cast the deciding vote in favor of the Wheaton group, was meeting the consultants for the first time. Absent were several prominent members of the steering committee, including Dr. Saltzman, Meredith Klein, and Blanche Reiner. Significantly, no one acknowledged the absence of the better part of the steering committee during the course of the meeting.

The NQWC representative called the meeting to order. Although this was the twenty-first meeting of the steering committee, the group still looked to him for leadership, so it was not considered odd that he assumed the responsibility of chairing the meeting. He gave a brief opening statement and turned the meeting over to Eric Moore, the designated on-site consultant of the Wheaton group.

In his long initial presentation, Moore stressed the importance of getting to know a lot more about Parkside as a system and Barnard 5 in particular. "We've got to develop a sense of trust toward one another" was the message throughout the meeting. A careful diagnostic approach would be the first step in realizing the project's dual objectives—the improvement of patient care and quality of working life on the nursing unit. Moore noted that the two objectives were interdependent and would be taken up concurrently.

As Moore spoke, his Parkside audience seemed interested in what was being said but offered few comments or indications of their feelings. The one notable expectation was Moe Kurtzman, who nodded enthusiastically at several of Moore's points. Kurtzman's energy was felt throughout the meeting, although he took a position that was not totally supportive of the project. On the one hand, Kurtzman pledged the union's full cooperation to Moore and the rest of the Wheaton team and proclaimed the importance of QWL for union members. The task force on Barnard 5 would provide a mechanism, he said, for helping to protect workers from annoying and sometimes dangerous conditions, such as needles that had been carelessly left around work areas by house physicians. He stated that he would make sure that the Wheaton consultants would not be confused with the team from Healthtech, the management consulting firm that had been hired by Harvey Hertz, the director of Parkside, to rationalize staffing patterns and improve productivity. From Kurtzman's perspective, the Healthtech team was there "to chop off heads."

But Kurtzman made it clear that because of his heavy schedule, he would not be able to attend many of the steering committee meetings; he would send an assistant in his place. His message was that he would back the project but that he also had more important things to be concerned about.

The meeting covered little substantive business. Its apparent purpose was to allow the principals from the different constituent groups an opportunity to get to know each other and to generate a spirit of goodwill that would help get things off on the right foot. It seemed to work. In fact, by the end of the meeting the expressions of mutual support were so strong that it was easy to overlook the absence of many of the key Parkside participants.

But the meeting also foreshadowed problems to come. At one point a steering committee member discounted Kurtzman's concerns about Healthtech and offered to arrange a meeting between Healthtech and Wheaton. None of the Wheaton consultants took up the offer, nor did anyone provide an acknowledgment that contact with Healthtech might pose a problem for Wheaton's relationship with the union. There was also a serious question about the commitment to the project on the part of both union and management. There were no members of the hospital's senior management group at the meeting except for Meredith Klein, who sat on the SMG as the representative from the nursing division. Harvey Hertz expressed no willingness to come to the meeting, and he sent no message of support. Instead, Hertz and the rest of the hospital's top administrators came under attack in absentia through Kurtzman's statement on Healthtech. The one unambiguous "management representative" at the meeting was Loretta Musial, the director of training and development. But Musial's position was marginal—so marginal, in fact that it was abolished several months later in a round of cost cutting.

There was no question that Moe Kurtzman was the legitimate representative of the Hospital Workers' Union. But his contradictory statements—first affirming union support for the Wheaton group and the goals of the project but later telling the group that he was too busy to remain a regular participant—indicated a real commitment problem as well. Sally McBride, the representative from the State Nurses' Association, remained silent throughout the meeting. This reflected perhaps her low profile work style but it also symbolized the weak reputation of the SNA in the hospital; when Parkside employees made a reference to "the union" it was in the singular and a clear reference to the Hospital Workers' Union.

The two representatives from the Barnard 5 Task Force, Bruce Gould and Nancy Baldwin, said little during the meeting. They faced a difficult and ambiguous situation. They were ultimately responsible for choosing Wheaton, insofar as the small working group on the unit made the final selection decision. But the group that clearly mattered was the project steering committee, not the Barnard 5 Task Force. Moreover, the relationship between the steering committee and the unit group had never been totally clarified. This issue was not addressed at all during the meeting.

Thus, while the meeting ended as hopefully as it began, with expressions of good will and the exchange of phone numbers between many of the participants, it was far from a satisfactory start. The project lacked a sense of direction. The steering committee and the unit task force were still not effective working groups that could function independently of the NQWC representative and provide a clear statement of their interests and needs to the consultant group. There was no discussion of specific action, nor was there a date set for the next steering committee meeting.

In the weeks that followed, Moore met individually with several members of the Barnard 5 staff as the first step in the diagnostic activity that he indicated would be the first stage of project activity. Moore also adopted the Columbia research team's method of participant observation; he spent a great deal of time walking about the nursing unit and watching the flow of work over the course of a shift. A few months before the Wheaton group was selected, one member of the Columbia team spent twenty-four continuous hours on the nursing unit in order to thoroughly become acquainted with the staff and their work. Moore thought this was a good idea and tried it himself. It made a difference. By the time the bleary-eyed Moore left the floor he had become a topic of conversation and had earned the respect and commitment of Barnard 5 staff. As the winter months passed, Moore continued his observations and interviews and began to collate employee opinions about quality of work life on the unit into an "issue census" that was intended as a basis for later action.

FIRST PROJECT SITE VISIT

The first major event in this early phase of consultant activity came at the end of February of 1976 in the form of a site visit from the project officer and the external review committee of the project's funding source, the Health Services Administration of the U.S. Department of Health, Education & Welfare. Since this was the initial site visit, it was regarded as extremely important, and considerable effort was devoted to the advance planning. Five steering committee members were selected for the panel that would represent the project. They were: Dr. Saltzman, Moe Kurtzman, Meredith Klein, Sally McBride, and Loretta Musial.

The five were referred to as "volunteers," but in reality they were chosen because they represented the major constituencies involved in the project. Early on the day of the site visit, the five met with the rest of the steering committee for a last minute briefing which included a report on Barnard 5 from Eric Moore. David Nadler of the Columbia team had given them a list of questions that might be asked of the group by the site visitors, and during this meeting, the steering committee delegation rehearsed their answers. The process was reminiscent of the consultant choice interviews except this time the group was on the receiving end of the questions. There were some awkward moments during the meeting as it became apparent that none of the steering committee members had a firm knowledge of what progress, if any, had been made in developing a viable task force on Barnard 5. But by the end of the meeting, the group had heard enough from Moore and two Barnard 5 staff members to assure itself that progress had been made.

The group's preparation paid off. During the course of a long afternoon, the HEW review team held private interviews and group meetings with the five steering committee representatives. At the end of the day, the HEW team told the Columbia research group (which, along with the consultants, had been excluded from most of the sessions) that things had gone very well. Their opinions were confirmed several weeks later when Dr. Saltzman received a letter from the HEW project monitor on behalf of the review team. The letter stated in part that:

All of us came away from the meeting with a high degree of enthusiasm and increased optimism about the likelihood of a successful outcome, especially considering the pressures of your work and the difficulties which are being faced by the Hospital as a whole.

The meeting was a high point in the early history of the steering committee. The group had demonstrated to itself and to the outside world that the Parkside Quality of Work Life Project was a legitimate, going concern. Group members felt a personal commitment to each other as well. On a number of occasions, Moe Kurtzman made testimonial-like statements about the changes in interpersonal relationships that had come about because of the project. Most centered on the attitudes of Dr. Saltzman.

Now Art knows that there are other people out there on the unit—my people. The doctors are going to learn that the housekeeper is part of the patient care team too.

The members of the committee were genuinely pleased and perhaps a bit surprised that an aggregation of individuals of varied backgrounds and who represented different and sometimes conflicting constituencies could become a cohesive, friendly group of people who enjoyed each other's company and treated each other with respect. Regardless of the other outcomes, the project seemed to add something to the quality of work life of the members of the steering committee.

Despite these interpersonal triumphs, the steering committee was still not an effective task-oriented group. Its major problem was an inability to define its role, particularly in relation to the Barnard 5 Task Force. Some steering committee members, including Moe Kurtzman, felt that changes suggested by the Barnard 5 group should be presented to the steering committee for approval. "It's important to keep the impact of the project in mind; otherwise, someone is bound to step on toes," Kurtzman said. It should be noted here that such jurisdictional concerns are often part of the history of quality of work life programs, especially during the early phases. In many cases the issue of the proper scope of a QWL program is expressed in terms of interference with the union contract. Indeed, most joint union-management QWL programs build a clause into the shelter agreement between the two parties which establishes the formal basis for QWL that under no circumstances should project activity infringe upon contractual matters, such as working hours, rates of pay, and job duties. Some projects do cross the boundary of what is contractual but it is always within the terms of a prior understanding that sanctions any specific contractual changes. Such matters are never taken casually.

It would appear, however, that the steering committee was not particularly concerned with possible contractual violations in wanting to limit the range of action of the unit-based working group. This was certainly true of Kurtzman. Like many militant union officials, he carried in his pocket a well-worn copy of the union's contract with management. He often boasted that he knew its complex provisions far better than his labor relations counterparts "across the table." But at no point did he invoke the sanctity of the contract in speaking of the need to keep the Barnard 5 group on a short tether. Rather, he was articulating the uncertainty the steering committee felt about its future role in the project. The committee had invested a great deal of time in the project, had turned over responsibility for selecting the project consultant to the fledgling Barnard 5 group (with disturbing results), and was not yet ready to delegate further responsibility. Perhaps if committee members had been clearer about their future status, they would have been more willing to allow the unit group to pursue its own agenda. At the steering committee meeting following the site visit, Kurtzman pointed out that the Barnard 5 group might suggest a change involving a patient care issue that should properly remain within the authority of the hospital's medical board. Seconding Kurtzman's point, Moore noted that the administration of the hospital also might want to place limits on the scope of task force activity. He told steering committee members that they were in a better position to have a broader and more realistic view of the whole Parkside system than task force participants, a statement that affirmed the view that Barnard 5 staff should avoid the big issues, at least initially.

But what *should* the unit task force be concerned with? The steering committee had no firm idea, but some of its members believed that the unit group should limit itself to small and manageable tasks, such as dealing with the problem of carelessly-placed needles. Since the source of this problem was house staff, Steering Committee members applauded Moore's suggestion (derived from his conversations with unit staff) that the Barnard working group should plan an orientation program for new doctors on the floor. Support for the idea was not unanimous: Sally McBride, the SNA representative, commented that "doctors will always be doctors"; her point was that physicians would never really be a part of the project since they are elitists and in an adversarial role in relation to everyone else.

The steering committee never did come to a decision about what the Barnard 5 Task Force should be doing, nor was the committee certain about how much control it should exert over the group to insure that staff members on the unit were not exceeding their authority. But at this point these issues did not seem critical since on the process side, things seemed to be working well. The committee had gained a large measure of confidence through its performance during the February site visit. There was enough trust among members that disagreements could be expressed openly without threatening the group's integrity. But it was also clear that the future of the project would be determined by what it actually did to improve the quality of work life and patient care and not by how well steering committee members got along among themselves. The focus of attention shifted naturally to Barnard 5 and Moore's attempts to form a viable working group among staff members. We will describe Moore's strategy but first, it is useful to provide a description of the pilot unit, Barnard 5.

BARNARD 5

Barnard 5 is a surgical nursing unit that occupies a floor of one of the hospital's older patient pavilions. In many ways, it is a typical nursing unit, and its problems are common to large tertiary care hospitals everywhere.

Coming off one of the two elevators that provide the main public entrance to the floor, a visitor faces the command center of the unit—the nursing station. To the immediate right of the elevators is a pay phone booth; the telephone is ostensibly for visitors, but it is used much more by staff to send and receive personal calls.

The nursing station is small and cramped. It is always busy. Nurses, nursing aides, unit clerks, off-floor personnel, and house staff work and "hang out" there. It is open on two sides: One opening faces the elevator lobby, the other leads on to the main corridor of the unit. Except for minor details, the nursing station could easily serve as the setting for a movie about a 1950 hospital. It looks and feels outdated. Nor is it a marvel of industrial engineering. The patient chart rack is kept right by the corridor opening; thus it is difficult to find, read, or replace charts without blocking movement to and from the corridor. Staff members continually bump into stools, chairs, and each other. As in work settings everywhere, the staff adds personal touches which serve to mask the bleakness of the setting—a couple of philodendron pots, post cards from vacationing colleagues and cartoons clipped from magazines.

On one side of the main corridor are seven four-person semiprivate rooms and a couple of single rooms that are used for patients who need special care or who are waiting for a bed in one of the sex-segregated semiprivate rooms. All are standard hospital rooms—neither cramped nor particularly inviting. Venetian blinds and the height of the window units severely restrict the patients' view to the outside. But noise from the intense street traffic is readily apparent. On the elevator and nursing station side of the corridor are several other rooms. Just behind the nursing station is the staff locker and wash room. At the end of the hall is the patients' lounge, a small, perpetually smoky room with institutional chairs and an out-of-focus black and white TV. The shabbiness of the room and the lack of recreational materials were the subject of frequent complaints from patients and staff alike.

In the other direction, there is a small kitchenette which is used for warming patient trays and for glassware. This is near the service elevator, which is used to transport supplies, patients to and from the operating room, and the bodies of patients who die on the unit. Beyond is the small resting room for house staff. At the end of the corridor is another private room.

The floor has little charm, but it is clean and functional. The corridor is kept relatively free of equipment, and there are never more than four patients to a room. These are conditions that would identify it as a nursing floor within a private voluntary hospital as opposed to one of the city's municipal hospitals.

At the time of the quality of work life project, there were twenty-six employees assigned to the unit (exclusive of the usual complement of five or six surgical residents). Half of the staff was on the day shift. The bulk of the staff was evenly divided between general duty RNs and nursing aides and assistants. (A nursing aide is eventually promoted to the level of nursing assistant, but there is little observable change in work responsibilities.) There is also one unit clerk on both day and evening shifts, a social worker (who covers another floor as well), and a head nurse on each of the three shifts. At Parkside the title of the latter has been upgraded to senior clinical nurse.

At the time of the project, Barnard 5 staff had a reputation for being energetic and committed to patient care. According to several staff members, Barnard 5 and a similar unit on the floor below are the most hectic of the pavilion's seven nursing units; this is due in large part to the severity of illnesses of the patients on Barnard 5. Many patients have cancer, including numerous cases of stomach cancer. Deaths on the unit are not infrequent. Colostomies (forming an artificial anal opening in the colon) and splenectomies are the most common types of operations performed.

There is tremendous variation in the nature and intensity of work on the unit over the course of a twenty-four hour period. Most patients are admitted to the unit on the evening shift. The unit clerk is responsible for assigning patients to beds. Sometimes there is no bed available; this means a temporary stay on another floor. No patient is refused entry unless all the beds in the hospital are full.

Barnard 5 operates at or near capacity at all times except for a brief period around the Christmas holidays. Most patients are admitted in the standard way—by the order of a Parkside attending physician—although a few are admitted through the emergency room. The unit handles about fifteen operations a week, and the average patient stay is about two weeks.

The busiest time of the daily cycle is in the morning. Morning rounds take place at about 7:00. The chief resident, accompanied by the other residents and one or two of the unit's nurses, moves from bed to bed, discussing medical aspects of each patient's condition. Grand rounds—led by an attending surgeon—are held every Wednesday. The rounds last about an hour. Most operations and transfers to clinical services such as radiology and nuclear medicine also take place in the morning. Throughout the morning, a constant stream of personnel comes onto the unit. These include residents, dietary workers, transporters who move patients to and from the floor and to clinical services departments and operating rooms located in other parts of the hospital, the messengers who pick up test specimens and deliver test reports, technicians with portable X-ray machines for patients who cannot be moved from the unit, housekeeping personnel, and nursing supervisors. Within the hospital context, a nursing unit such as Barnard 5 is the equivalent of a "shop floor," and one rarely sees representatives of upper levels of management from nursing or any of the other divisions.

In comparison with the day shift, the 3:30 to 11:30 evening shift is more relaxed. Evening rounds are held about 5:00 and tend to be more informal and shorter than morning rounds. The evening shift includes patient visiting hours. The hospital rule that limits patients to two visitors at a time is not strictly enforced, perhaps because at any given time it is unusual for more than five or six patients to have visitors. The afternoon hours are also given over to visits from attending physicians and the social worker assigned to the unit. It is also the time when many patients who have undergone an operation that morning are being returned from the postoperative recovery room.

For patients, the afternoon and evening hours are the most boring period of the day. The floor provides little in the way of recreational facilities apart from the drab TV lounge, so many of the patients kill time by walking up and down the corridor—many of them wheeling along portable IV stands. Members of the Columbia research team who were involved in participant observation on the unit were continually being asked what the weather was like "on the outside." Despite the relative freedom and the climate of boredom, one seldom hears conversations taking place between ambulatory patients. Most encounters are limited to a few words—a complaint about the brusqueness of the staff or how long it seems to take to get a nurse to the bedside. Patients seldom talk about their own medical condition, perhaps because for many, the prognosis ranges from serious to hopeless. Patients can often be traumatized by their operations; one nurse commented that colostomy patients often avoided looking at their protruding intestine.

The night shift is relatively relaxed. Staffing is reduced to either one or two RNs and a couple of nursing assistants. Patient contact is limited to the administration of scheduled medications to sleeping patients, comforting those who wake up in pain and making occasional rounds to insure that colostomy bags and IVs are in order. The rest of the time is spent in the nursing station doing paper work. The night shift is the only period when one could observe staff members with time on their hands, however briefly. But apart from these occasional night respites, the work is constant. However, from the observer's perspective, it appeared that RNs work at a considerably more intense pace than the nursing assistants, who sometimes resort to make-work—for example, straightening the arrangement of charts in the chart rack or recording patient temperatures with the deliberateness of a calligrapher. For RNs a lull in direct patient care functions means only one thing—an opportunity to catch up on required paperwork. Every change in the patient's condition must be logged in—every new IV bottle, every dose of medication. There is a separate, locked cabinet for narcotic drugs and a separate log for narcotics administration. By regulation, nurses are supposed to record a medication in the patient's chart at the time of administration. In practice, it is done when time allows.

The difference in the activity levels of nurses and nursing assistants is no doubt related to the scope of their job descriptions; there is only so much the assistant is allowed to do. But given the pressures placed upon them, it is easy to see how nurses come to interpret differential responsibilities in terms of motivation and character. To a lesser extent, a similar relationship holds for residents and nurses, although here the issue is more a matter of whether the nurse's duties are worthy of the claim to professional status. This hierarchy of disrespect between doctors and nurses and between nurses and the nonprofessional employees belies the official characterization of unit staff as the "patient care team."

THE EVOLUTION OF A CONSULTANT STRATEGY

As noted earlier, Moore began to visit Barnard 5 shortly after the January 9 steering committee meeting. He found a working group on the unit: the Barnard 5 Task Force, that had been brought together by the NQWC representative. Unlike the steering committee, the unit-based group lacked an identifiable membership. In theory, it included all of the twenty-six permanent staff members assigned to the three work shifts on the unit. In practice, the group consisted of a small core of the younger and higher status staff members and included several RNs, the senior clinical nurse on the day shift (Cathy Thomas), and the social worker whose responsibilities included the unit (Nancy Baldwin). All were day shift personnel. Initially at least, the only staff person from the evening shift to express an interest in the project was Ethel Atkins, the senior clinical nurse. Atkins—she was usually called by her last name as a sign of affection—was exceptional in a number of other ways. She was considerably older than the other active task force members, and she was the only active black member. Atkins commanded considerable respect on the unit, both for her clinical reputation and her interpersonal skills.

Notably absent in the early meetings with the NQWC representative and throughout the consultant selection period were the nonprofessional staff. These included nursing aides and assistants, licensed practical nurses, and the unit's housekeeper. After Moore arrived on the unit, a number of the nonprofessional staff members attended the meetings but usually sat off to the side, said little, and often drifted off before the termination of the meetings. In addition, the clerk on the day shift, a Hospital Workers' Union delegate, was hostile toward the project and despite the urgings of a number of staff members, was never enticed into becoming involved.

From early on, Moore faced significant structural problems in his attempts to form a viable working group—problems that often complicate administrative reform efforts in hospitals and other types of residential care facilities. The fact that staff were spread out over a three-shift, seven-day-a-week operation made it enormously difficult to schedule meetings. The night shift was all but impossible to bring into the formal task force structure. The highest staffing point was around 3:00 PM, the time of transition from the day to evening shift. But this time was reserved for the nurses' report—the main daily exchange of information on the condition and care plans of all patients on the unit. This was also visiting time, when nurses added policing duties to their patient care responsibilities.

The slack periods on the unit were the late mornings and early afternoons, and these were the times when most task force meetings were held. Occasionally, a 5:30 meeting would be scheduled on the afternoon shift. Staff members often had to come from home to attend meetings, and the hospital provided no compensation time. It was a tribute to the staff's commitment to change on the unit that many staff members did come in, even on their days off.

But apart from these problems of time and communication, the major issue was figuring out what to do. Improving patient care and quality of working life were certainly worthwhile goals, but how to translate them from abstractions to specific actions and plans was obvious to no one.

The product of Moore's interviews with Barnard 5 was a long list of problems that was similar to the problem census from the Columbia research group's baseline interviews carried out during the previous year prior to the initiation of the project. Moore's list offered no clues about where to start or what was a manageable problem. Throughout this period, Moore remained nondirective. His approach was to bring the staff together and ask them where they wanted to start. When a staff member would ask him about his opinion, he would turn the question around and direct it back to the questioner.

Gradually, the group began to show signs of uneasiness over how difficult it was to settle upon an initial focus for action. One nurse suggested that people might be afraid of expressing their true feelings. The process of bringing together staff members of different levels for the purpose of improving worklife was a concept foreign to Parkside. Perhaps, she said, things take more time than one expects and patience is the key. But Moore provided little assurance that things would eventually pick up. Instead, he offered procedural suggestions. He advised staff to go over the data that he and the Columbia group had collected and come up with some ideas for what they wanted to do. He also suggested attaching a box to the unit's bulletin board for people to put their ideas into (he avoided the term "sugestion box") and volunteered to type up incoming suggestions.

At one point, Moore decided that the task force should be restructured. He cited his problems in finding times to hold meetings and suggested that a supracommittee be formed—a committee of seven or eight members that would represent all levels of staff on the unit.

The proposal was not well received. One staff member commented that the plan was inefficient and that a newsletter might be a more effective way of conveying information. Another staff member discounted the idea of a representative committee on the grounds that "it would still be us." Several other ideas were proposed for improving the communication between shifts, but the staff was unable to come to an agreement on any basic plans for action. After his proposal was rejected, Moore appeared "very discouraged," according to Bruce Gould, the task force's informal leader. "We know that Eric is floundering" he added. Gould was also concerned about the decidedly management orientation of the Wheaton group. He commented that: "We are disturbed that Moore went to the hospital director before he came to see us. I thought he was supposed to work for us, that he was our consultant."

Nonetheless, by the spring of 1976, Barnard 5 staff had begun to identify some possible change projects. The most promising was the orientation program for new residents. Every three months, a new group of three or four residents came onto the unit, and this led to a number of predictable problems. The doctors had no idea where charts, medications and so forth were kept. They had to be continually informed about the normal operating procedures on the unit, and this often disrupted the work of unit staff. The members of the Barnard 5 Task Force felt that spending an hour or two with new residents when they started on the unit would make for a much smoother working relationship. Working independently of Moore, a small group began to develop some ideas for an orientation.

Unfortunately, the orientation project, like all other ideas that were suggested over the course of these first several months, never moved beyond the discussion phase. The group turned to the consultant for ideas and technical support but his response was invariably, "It's really up to you." The members of the task force became more discouraged by the week. Attendance at meetings held up; several people continued to come in on days off; but the tone of the meetings was often self-conscious, stiff, and ritualized. On one occasion, it seemed that staff members called a meeting for the benefit of a member of the Columbia research team who had come to the unit earlier in the day to confirm the time of a scheduled (but since forgotten) meeting. Moore never addressed the self-doubt and sense of unease that pervaded the Barnard working group. Instead, his response was to issue the following memorandum: (see Figure 5.1).

As far as the Columbia research team could determine, no one responded to Moore's memo, and the choice of a project was never made. Moore seemed to have disappeared from the floor, and by early May, the QWL program had virtually no presence on the unit apart from the scheduled observations of the Columbia group. Those who had been active participants were confused and disappointed, but for the rest of the staff of Barnard 5, the QWL program was simply one more abortive pilot project.

Ironically, there was a quality of work life project of sorts on Barnard 5 that had no relationship to the official project. Since February, Ethel Atkins, the senior clinical nurse on the evening shift, had been holding staff meetings that focused on improving communication among staff members and on patient-based teaching. The group began to select patients as teaching cases and followed them through from admission to discharge. Evening staff members were openly enthusiastic about the meetings. They were a forum for resolving disputes and expressing feelings, and they allowed the nurses the opportunity to think reflectively about their professional responsibilities in a setting that was insulated from the hectic, task-oriented environment of the nursing floor. Atkins came up with the idea for the meetings herself. She viewed them as a natural outgrowth of her new role as senior clinical nurse of the evening shift. (In early 1976, the "head nurse" position had been upgraded as part of the reorganization of the nursing department.) Atkins attended a few of the official QWL meetings, but neither she nor anyone else suggested integrating her work with that of the Barnard 5 Task Force.

By early May, the Columbia team and staff from the National Quality of Work Center had concluded that the Wheaton intervention had failed. But officially, the decision to terminate Wheaton could only be made by the client—the project steering committee. Therefore, the two principal outside groups remained neutral and offered no opinion on the competence or future of the consulting group. Parkside participants were unsure of what to do. From the perspective of the unit, there was no existing project. The steering committee, however, seemed unaware of the total absence of activity on the unit and probably believed that as long as there was a project steering committee, there was a project. No one wanted to blame Moore. He was seen as ineffectual but also as a "nice guy." The other members of the Wheaton

Wheaton Associates

Memorandum

To: Barnard 5 Staff
From: Eric Moore, Quality of Work Life Project Consultant
Subject: Let's Get Moving

It has come time to select those projects to which you feel the Barnard 5 quality of work life project should direct its energies. Listed below are five potential projects related to issues identified through the diagnostic process. All of these projects will require your further participation in providing information, developing action plans and evaluating results.

Please rank the listed projects in terms of which you would like to see tackled first: Put a 1 next to the project you consider most important, a 2 next to the one you would consider second most important, . . . and so on. Then put this sheet in a sealed envelope and leave it with your elected Chairperson.

Wheaton Associates   **Attachment**
Barnard 5 Quality of Work Life Project

Rank

( )   A.   Develop a program for introducing new residents to Barnard 5.

                This program would be directed at reducing some of the quality of work life and patient care problems associated with new residents coming onto the service. It would probably involve the preparation of some form of written "guide book" containing information that would be helpful for a new resident to know. It would also involve the selection of representatives from all permanent staff groups, who would each prepare a short oral briefing on how their group fits into the total patient care picture of Barnard 5. This would be presented to the new residents prior to, or within, the first few days of their arrival on the floor.

( )   B.   Initiate a study of nursing staff scheduling practices.

                This study would be directed at examining current practices in nursing staff scheduling with the objective of discovering ways in which such scheduling might be changed in order to improve both the quality of work life and the delivery of patient care.

( )   C.   Initiate a study of the frequency and effects of late patient admissions on Barnard 5 operations.

                This study would be directed at examining how frequently late admissions occur and what effects such admissions have on the quality of work life for the staff and the delivery of patient care.

( )   D.   Develop a method to register and process complaints.

                This would involve development of a formalized system to bring up and deal with staff complaints related to the quality of work life or patient care.

( )   E.   Establish priorities for various work assignments to be carried out under different staffing conditions.

                This project would be directed at determining the priority of the various work activities carried out by the nursing staff. It would provide guidelines as to what activities each member of a shift would emphasize or deemphasize, depending upon the overall number of available staff members.

Figure 5.1

team were not viewed as kindly, but they were on Barnard 5 only rarely and attended few steering committee meetings.

The malaise dragged on through the spring of 1976. The Wheaton group brought in an interpersonal specialist to work with Moore on the unit. The new consultant, like Moore, failed to generate a focused action plan for the unit, although plans for the doctor's orientation continued. Unlike Moore, he was disliked by practically everyone, so after a number of unsuccessful meetings, Moore was alone once again.

The strained atmosphere throughout this period is illustrated in the following exchange between Moore and members of the task force.

BRUCE GOULD (to Moore): "How do we work on this doctors' orientation? I don't know how to work on such a problem." Turning to Moore, Gould continues, "When you wrote this item on your list (of possible projects), did you have anything in mind?"

MOORE: "How do you deal with a problem like this? What do you want to accomplish by doing this? You're going to have to deal with these issues as part of this process. Did you pick this because it was the easiest project to do?"

GOULD: "No. We picked it because it was something concrete."

Silence.

MOORE: "What do you hope to accomplish?"

Silence.

Then Cathy Thomas, the day shift senior clinical nurse, answers: "We would like to have a cleaner unit where we're not always picking up after the doctors. We want better communication, and we want to reduce the frustration of the nurses."

MOORE: "What will happen?"

GOULD: "It will be a joke."

MOORE: "What do you do to make them (the doctors) take it seriously?"

There is another period of silence. Then, Moore turns to Jerome Walker, a nursing aide who has been sitting silently in the corner since the meeting began.

MOORE says: "What do you think?"

WALKER: "What do I think about what?"

MOORE: "What should we be doing on the unit?"

WALKER: "I don't have anything to say."

MOORE: "You like the way things are here? Nothing on this list
             is important to you?"
WALKER: "It's all important. But I want to see results. When
             something starts happening, then I'll have something
             to say. Until then I have nothing to say."
GOULD   (to Walker): "Things are improving on the ward, aren't
             they?"
WALKER: "I'm really tired. I'd rather not talk."

THE DISMISSAL OF THE WHEATON GROUP

In early June, the Hospital Workers' Union went on strike at Parkside
and several other hospitals in the city. By mutual agreement, all QWL
project activity was suspended for the duration of the strike. Following
the strike's settlement eight days later, the Columbia group resumed
its observations on Barnard 5. On several occasions, the research team
was asked: "Where is Eric?" "Is he coming back?" As far as anyone
could tell, Moore had stopped coming to the floor in early April, and his
last communication to the unit was his April 30 memo exhorting the
staff to "get moving." Effectively, there was no longer a quality of work
life project on Barnard 5.

The first official project event following the settlement of the strike
was a meeting of the steering committee on June 18. The principal
agenda item was a request from Art Dowling of the Wheaton team to
take a group of Barnard 5 staff members off the unit for two days in
order to plan a major activity that was "in the works." After Dowling
presented the plan there was, at first, little response. Then a cascade of
criticisms were voiced. Moe Kurtzman warned that the chronic
staffing problem made it extremely difficult to pull staff from the floor.
Blanche Reiner asked Dowling, "*You* feel the need for this time, but
what about the steering committee?" The meeting ended with no
formal decision made about the Wheaton proposal. Leaving the room,
Reiner remarked in a public voice, "*I still* have deep reservations about
those consultants." After the meeting Bruce Gould commented to a
member of the Columbia research team that he had no idea that
Dowling would propose a two-day off-site activity; indeed, no such plan
had ever been discussed on the floor. Dowling himself had virtually no
previous contact with the members of the task force on the nursing
unit. Gould also felt that the steering committee had very little idea
about the status of the project on Barnard 5.

The June 18 meeting marked the beginning of the end of the
Wheaton group's tenure. The fact that by suggesting the off-site pro-

gram the consultants had violated an earlier understanding that project activity must take place within normal working hours provided the immediate rationale for dismissal. But the general feeling was summed up by Blanche Reiner: "We all agree that they are no good."

Again, the steering committee could not bring itself to take decisive action and left the decision to fire Wheaton up to a vote of the Barnard 5 Task Force. Four weeks later, the unit group met and voted to dismiss the Wheaton team. On August 6, the steering committee met for the thirtieth time since the initial meeting in May of 1975 and ratified the Barnard 5 Task Force's decision. The steering committee authorized the National Quality of Work Center representative to draft a letter of termination to Wheaton Associates. Moving on, the steering committee began to lay down some guidelines for the selection of a new project consultant.

INTERPRETIVE SUMMARY: THE QUALITY OF WORK LIFE PROJECT AT THE END OF THE WHEATON ASSOCIATES PERIOD

There were, in effect, two quality of work life projects at Parkside. The first came to an end with the dismissal of the Wheaton Associates consulting team in August of 1976; the second began a month later with the selection of Bill Evans and Associates as the new project consultant. Although most of this narrative will be devoted to describing and assessing the project subsequent to the hiring of the Evans group, it is useful here to assess the factors that led to the failure of Wheaton Associates and to comment on the impact of the Wheaton period on the QWL project at Parkside.

There were at least three factors that were crucial in the dismissal of the Wheaton Associates group. First, there were unresolved problems left over from the consultant selection phase of the project, particularly the failure to develop viable groups within the hospital. Secondly, much of the failure has to be attributed to the lack of competence and what must be regarded as a certain degree of bad faith on the part of the Wheaton Associates group. The third factor was the inability of the Quality of Work Life Project Steering Committee to take decisive action once evidence began to accumulate that the project was faltering.

Each of these factors will be discussed in turn. The data on which the following account is based were derived from participant observation as well as intensive interviews with principal figures involved in the project during this early phase of its history.

The Consultant Selection Process

One of the most serious shortcomings of the QWL project in its early phases was the inability of the steering committee to act as a viable client. This in turn is partially attributable to the failure of the sponsoring groups, the Institute for Social Research and the National Quality of Work Center, to present the steering committee with a clear picture of what the project was about and what the consultant group was supposed to do. The steering committee remained heavily dependent on the NQWC representative in the months after the initial union-management meeting in May of 1975. The group never became an autonomous, proactive, decision-making body. Moreover, its membership was never stabilized. As news of the project spread, new people would join the group. Some remained, but others would attend one or two meetings and then drop out. Also, the project was never able to find a permanent representative from the Parkside Residents' Committee. This was due partly to the decertification of PRC, which eliminated its official standing in the project, and partly to the transient nature of the hospital residency. The movement of staff in and out of the steering committee made it difficult to evolve norms governing attendance, and it limited the development of trust among participants.

In hindsight, many of the problems described here were common to many "first generation" QWL programs. In more recent programs, considerable attention is devoted to the training of steering committee members—providing them with essential group and interpersonal skills, and conveying a realistic sense of what will be expected of them. Many consultants provide "facilitator" training, whereby selected union and management representatives on the steering committee learn skills that will enable them to take on the responsibilities of the external consultant team after it has left the site. Such training takes place well before the intervention stage of the QWL program begins. The consequences of the failure to provide these types of early entry training at Parkside are very clear: After several months and an intensive schedule of meetings, the steering committee still did not have a sense of what it was supposed to do.

Another key problem was the protracted length of the consultant selection period. While this period provided a vehicle for participants to get to know one another, it did not help to clarify what the labor-management group wanted from the consultants on the project, and valuable energy was lost. In the end, the ultimate consultant choice was accidental. It would have been useful to have devoted more time to building a sense of the goals of the project, a sense of ownership, an idea of what participants had to gain from the project. Had the steering committee known what it wanted, the choice of a consultant group would probably have been more informed; it also may have been less time consuming. Again the importance of providing training to participants *before* the initiation of the action phase of the project must be emphasized.

The hasty decision to leave the final selection to the Barnard staff could either be interpreted as a means of eliciting bottom-up participation or an attempt to avoid the consequences of a faulty decision. In retrospect, the evidence seems to favor the latter interpretation. By the time the consultant selection process had been narrowed down to the final three groups, there was, in reality, still no viable, cohesive project task force on the nursing unit. This is another example of the need for early training of key participants. Responsibility for developing a working group on Barnard 5 fell to the NQWC representative. He functioned well in bringing unions and management to the table and working out an agreed-upon set of project goals. But he lacked experience in behavioral science theory and techniques and the skills necessary for moving the steering committee from an aggregation of voluntary participants with potentially common interests to a viable, committed, task-oriented group. Moreover, he lacked certain interpersonal skills which led the steering committee to not trust him. This distrust eventually included the project as a whole.

The Lack of Consultant Competence and Commitment to the Project

Moore was never able to effectively harness the considerable desire for change among Barnard 5 staff. He did not provide leadership, nor did he build the skills of Barnard 5 staff members. At most, he helped the staff to articulate previously unspoken grievances. What remains difficult to explain is Moore's long absences from the pilot unit. Throughout much of the Wheaton Associates period, the Columbia research team, which was involved in carrying out randomized time observations, provided the only outside presence on the experimental unit.

Another serious problem was Moore's isolation; there was never a functioning consultant team present in the hospital on an ongoing basis. Moore was the only consultant with "hands on" experience in the quality of work life project. Two of the other official members of the team—Dowling and Weinglass—spent practically no time on the site apart from meetings with the steering committee and with management principals in the hospital. The fourth team member, Carl Goode, was transferred to another city shortly after the project began and thus had no real involvement with the project. Only at the end of their tenure in the hospital did the Wheaton group assign a second on-site consultant. This individual arrived on the unit too late to have much of an impact other than provoking the hostility of staff members because of an overbearing personal style.

It should be noted that the Wheaton group had little previous experience in working with joint labor-management committees. From early on, the group was hindered by its reputation for having a "management orientation." The reputation seemed well founded. Following the development of the team's preliminary intervention plan during the last week of March, the team took their plan first to the hospital director and the vice president for personnel. They received approval from these two before they ever presented the plan to the Barnard 5 Task Force or the project steering committee. Despite the emerging union-management conflict over Healthtech Associates, the Wheaton group proposed to use Healthtech as part of its work on Barnard 5. And the Wheaton consultants proposed several briefings for hospital management but not a single briefing for union officials. In the group's April 6 meeting with Hospital Director Harvey Hertz, Art Dowling commented that, "Our perspective is basically one of a management consultating firm—we are used to working with and for management." If one assumes that the members of the Wheaton group were generally competent—and their previous reputations would support this assumption—then perhaps working jointly with unions and management demands a special set of skills and experience.

The Inability of the Steering Committee to Take Decisive Action against the Wheaton Group

Concerns about the lack of competence of the Wheaton group were being expressed openly by members of the Barnard 5 Task Force in early April of 1976. The steering committee did not take a vote to terminate the consultants until August 6 and then sent the results of the vote to the Barnard 5 group for the final decision. The letter of termination was sent to Wheaton on August 10. Thus the process lasted for four months. Why did it take so long?

This protracted denouement reflected the lack of goals and direction of the labor-management group. The steering committee wanted the project to continue, but it feared the consequences of firing the consultant group. Several members stated explicitly that they did not want to interview several consultant candidates all over again. As in the initial consultant selection phase, the group became heavily dependent on outsiders. The NQWC representative reemerged as a force within the committee meetings. Edward Lawler from ISR supplied the list of evaluation criteria used to assess the performance of the Wheaton group since it was clear to the members of the Columbia research team that the steering committee was not capable of carrying out an independent hearing on its own. It is significant to note that the process by which the Wheaton group was fired was in many ways similar to that in which the group was selected. Both required several meetings over a protracted time period and the substantial involvement of the outside groups. In both cases, the steering committee left the final decision to the working group on Barnard 5. Moreover, as in the initial consultant selection, only a handful of unit staff members was involved in the determining vote on the fate of the consultant group.

ASSESSMENT

It is difficult to evaluate the long-term impact of the Wheaton debacle on the quality of work life project at Parkside. The consultant group did not provide the Columbia research group with explicit criteria for project success. Therefore it was impossible to design a plan for measuring project outcomes. But the following conclusions seem warranted on the basis of the observational and interview data.

The project resulted in no significant changes in working life on the experimental unit, Barnard 5. The one identified action objective—the orientation program for new house staff—was still in the planning stage when the Wheaton group left the hospital.

The project did survive. The steering committee's major theme at this point was: "We've learned from our mistakes." The difficult dismissal process did not create serious conflict within the committee. All expressed a willingness to reset the clock and begin anew.

As described in the following chapter, the selection of the Evans group as the project consultant was remarkably tidier than the selection process for Wheaton. This could be interpreted as a sign of the growing competence of the steering committee.

The most serious damage resulting from the Wheaton period was perhaps the negative impact on Barnard 5 staff. Many of the staff members who were very involved in project meetings during the unit group's early days were considerably less active in the reconstituted project after the selection of the Evans consulting group. The Evans group took over as project consultants with about a fourth of the consultant budget exhausted. This made it necessary for the group to carefully ration its time, particularly toward the end of the project.

CHAPTER SIX

A New Beginning
The Early Stages of the Evans Consultation

The dismissal of the Wheaton group took place in early August, at the beginning of the hospital's peak vacation period. Throughout the rest of the month there was little project activity—in part because of the absence of several members of the steering committee but also because many felt the need for a respite from the project. A month's hiatus provided necessary separation between a sorry chapter that had finally come to an end and a hopeful new beginning for the project. David Nadler and Edward Lawler sensed that the steering committee did not want to repeat the lengthy consultant selection process and offered to provide the names and supporting materials of two or three qualified consultant groups for the committee's consideration. The group accepted the proposal without hesitation.

On September 8, the steering committee and representatives of the Barnard 5 group met to interview the consultant teams that had been selected by Lawler and Nadler. Sixteen months had elapsed since the initial union-management meeting, and the steering committee was coming together for the thirty-second time. For the first consultant selection round, the steering committee had devised an elaborate, almost ritualistic interviewing procedure. This time the group went about the task in a much more natural, straightforward way. Through its difficulties the committee had learned how to be a more demanding and competent client, and was in a far better position to make an informed choice than it had been in the fall of 1975.

The first group to be interviewed was the team headed by Bill Evans, one of the finalists in the previous round. The team was introduced, and its four members—Bill Evans, Steve Meyer, Dan Hartman, and Ron Hodges—briefly summarized their credentials. Their style was friendly and rather informal especially in contrast to the Wheaton Associates group. In his opening remarks, Ron Hodges cited some previous antiunion consulting work which drew a frown from Moe Kurtzman. But after this initial incident, there were no problems; by the end of an hour-long interview session, Kurtzman was a strong supporter of the Evans team.

Blanche Reiner started the more focused discussion of the Evans team's intended strategy for the project by asking: "I still don't know how things work with consultants. What are you going to do?" The consultants had been briefed thoroughly on the course of the project up to this point, and they were well aware of the Wheaton group's failure to generate any momentum. They also knew that the steering committee was desperate to get some quick results that would justify the continuance of the project and were quite willing to let the consultants "run with the ball."

Taking the cue, Dan Hartman walked over to the flip chart that the group had brought along and began what was clearly a well-prepared presentation. "We've been here three times now," he said. "We've thought a lot about this project. We've worked out some objectives." Hartman carefully described the overall goal of the proposed intervention—to help hospital personnel by providing problem-solving, communications, and conflict resolution skills. In the Evans plan, the steering committee would be the change agent for the total Parkside system and would be responsible for the diffusion of key ideas and innovations. Despite some differences in terminology, Hartman's sketch of a revitalized steering committee was strongly reminiscent of David Nadler's "hub of the wheel" image in the formative period of the group. Hartman spoke well; the Parkside group listened intently and appeared to be very pleased with what they heard. They were especially happy with the Evans team's affirmation that the consultants would be there when needed. As the consultant group left the room Kurtzman remarked: "No doubt about it. They are much better this time around."

The second consulting team, which was interviewed after the lunch break, had not been a candidate in the first selection round. Only three of the members of the proposed five member team were present. Of the other two, one was in Geneva and the other was in Australia. This prompted Moe Kurtzman to turn to Edward Lawler of ISR and say audibly: "What's he doing, chasing kangaroos?" Having provoked the steering committee's fear of the "no-show consultant," the group did little to recoup its losses. Indeed, despite outstanding academic reputations and considerable health care consulting experience, the consultants were remarkably inept at presentation skills. The three spent many tedious minutes presenting their credentials but provided little sense of what they would actually do at Parkside. They relied heavily on jargon, even after it was obvious from the blank expressions of steering committee members that "OD," "process consultation," and the like were essentially foreign terms. Then it became apparent that two of the three members of the group had never worked together—in fact, it wasn't clear that they had even met before the presentation. The consultants were trapped in a vicious circle in which nothing seemed to work, including humor. Kurtzman turned to one member of the team and said pointedly:

> None of you is locally based. And this is a twenty-four hour operation. You live three hundred miles from here (in a small town). How are you going to deal with the distance problem?

The consultant responded with an unsatisfactory answer and ended by joking that "I live so far away because that eliminates the parking problem." No one laughed. Dr. Saltzman commented disapprovingly: "It's hard enough for me to get in here from the suburbs."

The ensuing vote was predictably lopsided: Ten of the twelve votes were cast for Evans. One of the other group's two supporters was Ivan Edwards, the newly appointed clinical supervisor for Barnard 5. Edwards, who is black, noted that the presence of a black member on this team was an important consideration in view of the salience of race and status issues within the hospital. The other vote came from Nancy Marullo, the new assistant director of nursing for Barnard Pavilion and Edwards' supervisor. From her comments, it appeared that her vote was based on agreement with Edwards' position.

After the vote, the steering committee took up the issues Edwards has raised. The group noted that the Wheaton Associates team failed to reach out to the predominantly black nonprofessional staff—particularly, nursing aides and assistants and housekeeping personnel. But working on its own, the Barnard 5 Task Force had begun to bring these groups into project activities. Bruce Gould commented that: "Housekeeping has a change of attitude—they feel more involved now." The steering committee praised the Barnard group for its efforts and pledged that the Evans team would be sensitized to the race and class issues on the nursing unit. The committee would make sure that the consultants made special efforts to involve lower level staff in project activities. Edwards concluded what had been a remarkably frank and mature group discussion by saying that while he had not voted for the Evans team, he could certainly live with them. Edward Lawler added a coda: "You should tell Evans about your misgivings about them. They must know where you stand and what you want from them."

GETTING STARTED

Above all, the steering committee wanted quick action on Barnard 5. If the task force fell apart, it would be difficult to mobilize a new constituency for the project. Evans told the steering committee that he and his colleagues would not be able to establish an intensive presence on Barnard 5 until they had cleared their agendas of some longstanding commitments elsewhere. And unfortunately one of the team members, Ron Hodges, had to bow out from the project. The steering committee heard and accepted this, but Evans' candor and his promise to start as quickly as possible were not enough to eliminate the Parkside group's disappointment or its fear that the newly hired consultant team was treading the same path as Wheaton.

Some staff members were especially impatient. Two weeks after the September 8 meeting, Nancy Marullo approached one of the members of the Columbia research team. She said that she and her subordinate, Ivan Edwards, had gotten hold of Eric Moore's Problems and Priorities List and were about "to get to work on it before Evans arrives." This was the first of a series of occasions in which Marullo upstaged the Barnard 5 Task Force and the consultants, and it created a risk that the QWL project would become too identified with the supervisory staff of the nursing department.

There were other reasons for concern. Morale throughout Barnard Pavilion had reached a new low because of staff shortages caused by the hospital's tight financial situation. Understaffing led to a great deal of overtime and unscheduled weekend duty. It was not uncommon for general duty nurses, many of whom had young children, to find out an hour or two before their shift ended that a staffing emergency required them to stay on for two or three extra hours or, in some cases, another shift. Inevitably, deteriorating working conditions led to turnover: Several of the key RNs, who provided needed energy for the project in its early days, had either left the unit or were scheduled to leave within a few months.

Thus, following its selection by the project steering committee but prior to full-scale intervention activity on Barnard 5, the Evans consulting group found itself in this position: It enjoyed the trust and commitment of the steering committee, but no demands had ever been placed on the committee that would have required it to commit resources to a specific change project on Barnard 5 or elsewhere in the hospital. Staff morale on the experimental unit was at a low point. Labor-management relations at Parkside were entering a particularly troublesome period because of the hospital's difficult fiscal situation. The prospects for physician involvement seemed even more distant in the wake of NLRB decertification of the Parkside Residents' Committee. Moreover, the Evans group knew that it was starting out with about a quarter of the budgeted consultant funds already spent. It was not an ideal consulting situation.

In early October Evans, Meyer, and Hartman interviewed several staff members on Barnard 5 and held meetings on all three shifts to introduce themselves and identify problems that might provide a focus for later action. An outcome of the meetings was a task list which was divided into two categories. First, there were issues that Barnard 5 staff members could initiate and handle on their own, such as staff conferences and the proposed orientation for new residents. Second, there were issues that would necessarily involve key personnel at higher administrative levels in other sections of the hospital. A change in procedures for transporting patients from the floor to the radiology department, for example, would require the approval of medical and administrative personnel from radiology and, quite possibly, approval from the hospital's medical board. Evans made it clear to Barnard 5 staff that the unit group, not the consultants, would be responsible for choosing possible action projects but that the consultants would be available as facilitators who would assist unit staff in clarifying goals. The Evans team's approach was low key and nondirective; the group also conveyed a self-assurance and sense of caring that were conspicuously absent during Moore's tenure on the floor.

From the beginning, the consultants saw that working with Marullo and Edwards was not going to be easy. Neither was very popular with staff members, and any project activities that were closely identified with them would not be well received. Still, Evans and his colleagues believed that the two must be central to any serious change strategy, since Barnard 5 staff members were not in a position to implement successful innovations beyond the boundaries of the nursing unit. Marullo was enthusiastic about the QWL project, and she clearly enjoyed the attention she was receiving from the consultants; in return, she had nothing but praise for Evans at steering committee meetings. But her lack of focus was a major problem. As Meyer put it: "Nancy is moving in all sorts of directions at once." Helping her to clarify her role would be a major priority. The consultants' strategy for Edwards was different; they were concerned with his apparent unwillingness to exert his authority on Barnard 5. Thus efforts would be made to improve his leadership capabilities.

The Initial Evans Organizational Development Plan

In mid-October, the Evans group put forth their initial plan for the Barnard 5 project. (The text of the plan is included in the Appendix.) The overall objective described in the plan was to improve health care delivery and quality of working life on the experimental unit. Specific activities would include: developing health care improvement teams on Barnard 5; training individuals on the unit in problem solving and group work techniques; establishing a better communication link between the nursing unit and the steering committee; and developing the latter as the vehicle for the diffusion of organizational improvements coming out of project activity on Barnard 5. The organizational development (OD) plan followed a conventional action research sequence—entry and diagnosis, issue identification, planning, intervention activities, and the eventual termination of consultant involvement. Apart from the references to training Barnard 5 staff members and team development, the plan contained no details about what areas of group or organizational functioning the Evans team intended to change. Actual, specific changes would flow out of the diagnostic work and in collaboration with the client system.

Barnard 5 would continue to be the project's focal point, and the Evans plan reaffirmed the steering committee as the chief executive body of the project. The timetable called for an initial six-month period in which improvement targets would be identified. Implementation of at least some of the proposed action steps would begin during the fourth month. Diffusion of change processes to the larger Parkside system would begin after nine months and would continue to the end of the eighteen-month project period. Consistent with the philosophy of organizational development, the Evans plan concluded by saying, "Our improvement strategy is intended to leave the client system with the capability of maintaining the organizational improvement changes."

At this early point in the intervention, the Evans team had made substantial progress in eliminating the strong residue of apathy and mistrust that had been left by Wheaton. And the new team had a plan. The fact that it had a rather unspecific "off the shelf" quality to it mattered less than the fact that a working document was promised and produced—on time. But the group was also becoming aware of impediments that would persist throughout the entire course of the project. First, the potential for change on Barnard 5 was limited. Unit staff had little decision-making authority. Any meaningful change would almost certainly have to involve supervisory staff from outside the unit. The consultants recognized this and began to work on improving the leadership capabilities of nursing management within Barnard Pavilion. But this took precious time away from team-building efforts and other activities on Barnard 5.

Moreover, the Evans team members were coming to realize that the steering committee was not an effective policy-making group. Some of the more vocal members of the committee, such as Blanche Reiner, represented a hospital department with little influence over important administrative decisions. Reiner appointed an aide to the committee—a social service administrator who had no real connection to Barnard 5; she also said little at steering committee meetings. Still, she came to the meetings on a more regular basis than most members, despite the fact that it wasn't clear why she was there. Some of the more powerful members of the committee—notably, Meredith Klein, the director of nursing—seemed unwilling to commit resources to the quality of work life project or to make a strong public statement of support.

The most telling sign of the essential weakness of the steering committee was the absence of any other member of the hospital's seven person senior management group, apart from Meredith Klein. Harvey Hertz, the hospital director, continued to ignore the project. Neither Hertz nor Klein made any attempt to divert the Healthtech team away from Barnard 5. Not only did this disrupt the Evans group's efforts to build linkages with the Hospital Workers' Union and its nonprofessional class members, but it provided an embarrassingly clear sign of the low status of the project. How low became clear when Evans was compelled to interview an administrative intern in order to get management's view of the project—an indication of Evans' outsider position. Evans was told that the QWL project had "priority status" in the project management grid devised by the hospital's director of planning and management information systems. Unfortunately, it was one of the 143 such projects at Parkside.

HWU's commitment to the project was also questionable, despite the union's verbal enthusiasm at the time of the initial contacts with NQWC staff. The word from "downtown" (the term used to describe the union's headquarters) was that the QWL project was "Moe's boondoggle." The union saw it as basically a management-dominated project but one that posed few obvious dangers. One popular, cynical view was

that HWU tolerated the project because the union had acquired a reputation for being much more concerned about pay raises than patient
care, and the Parkside experiment provided good public relations.

If Kurtzman lacked the support of his superiors, he also had little
influence on Barnard 5. As the union's sole organizer for nonprofessional staff throughout the hospital, Kurtzman represented nearly
2000 employees. The nature of his position meant that employees he
knew well were limited to those who held an official position in the
union and those whom he represented in the grievance process. His fa-
miliarity with Barnard 5 and its staff was extremely limited. Moreover, he was a white male, and the great majority of HWU members on
the unit were black and Hispanic women. There was one union delegate on the floor, a unit clerk who had no use for the quality of work
life project and refused to participate in meetings or data-gathering activities. And she and Kurtzman were not on good terms. Her resistance
to the project was not critical, since she was not well-liked by many
staff members and had limited personal influence; but the unit clerk is
the nexus of information flow to and from the unit, and a supportive
person in this role would have made it easier for the project to address
the key unit problems identified in the earlier diagnoses.

Moe Kurtzman's behavior during these early months of the Evans
intervention merits some attention. He alternated between threatening to "pull the plug" on the project by withdrawing union support and
praising the Evans group for their efforts to bring a long overdue
measure of respect to "my people," as Kurtzman called HWU members. But as fall gave way to winter, he stopped coming to steering
committee meetings. At first, other committee members viewed this as
simple lack of interest. The prevailing interpretation was that despite
his grandstanding, Kurtzman didn't have much real commitment to
the process of collaborative change. Often, he was forgotten. But then,
sometimes without warning, Kurtzman, communicating through the
consultants, would become overtly hostile to the committee. He frequently accused management of packing the committee. Gradually,
his absence from steering committee meetings took on the meaning of
an active boycott. The steering committee became increasingly
unsympathetic to Kurtzman. In describing him, several members used
the image of a small child who throws a tantrum when he doesn't get
his way. But they also knew that Kurtzman had the power to back up
his threats: A Hospital Worker's Union pull-out would undoubtedly
have meant the end of external funding support. The project might suf-
fer from Kurtzman's histrionics, but without him, there would be no
project.

In retrospect, however, one loses some of the meaning of Kurtzman's stormy behavior by limiting it to the interpersonal level. Kurtzman was a "man in the middle," and his ambivalence reflected the strains inherent in his position. He was a skilled political operator who saw that the union had little enthusiasm for the project. By reputation, the Hospital Workers' Union was strong, hierarchical, and authoritarian. It delivered the goods at contract time and fought hard for its members in grievance proceedings, but it was never seen as a model of participatory democracy. One seasoned observer of the union suggested that it felt threatened by a venture that had as a goal the empowerment of lower level employees, most of whom were outside the union's delegate structure. Kurtzman knew that there was little to be gained by making a strong show of support for the project, and his posturing allowed him to keep a safe distance.

But there is also the question of why Kurtzman never followed through on his pull-out threat. Again, the political dimension must be considered. If HWU officially terminated its relationship with the project, it would have been interpreted as a sign of the union's bad faith and would have meant negative publicity. Because of Parkside's prominence and the unique coalition of interests involved, the project had won substantial recognition. But a more compelling reason was that Kurtzman genuinely liked and trusted Bill Evans. He felt that Evans understood the needs of the poorly-educated, low status men and women who carried out much of the tedious, unglamourous work on patient care units—such as lifting patients out of and into beds and washing floors. He viewed Evans as a sympathetic neutral, someone who wouldn't be conned by management's tricks. Kurtzman clearly liked the attention he received from the consultants, the research team, and, in less troubled times, his colleagues on the steering committee. And despite the headaches, the Parkside project enhanced Kurtzman's own stature in the hospital.

Thus at the end of the two-month entry and diagnostic period described in the organization development plan, Evans, Meyer, and Hartman still lacked strong support from both management and the principal union in the hospital. So they decided to intensify their focus on Barnard 5 in the hopes that a bottom-up strategy would produce results that would eventually gain higher recognition. Their diagnostic work reactivated some enthusiasm for the project among unit staff, although such support was still limited largely to the small core of young, day shift nurses who took an early interest in the philosophy of QWL. But the potential for wider involvement was there. Evans and Meyer—the two team members who worked on the unit—earned a reputation for being sympathetic, competent, and available. What was needed was a focus for activity. Jointly, the consultants and the Barnard 5 group decided to begin with two of the projects that had been suggested by staff members during the Wheaton period. These were: the monthly orientation meeting for new surgical residents and the weekly shift-based staff conferences.

The purpose of the residents' orientation was to provide new doctors with practical information on the layout of the nursing unit, work procedures, and supplies. The considerable physical variation among Parkside's nursing units created much confusion among rotating staff members who had to learn new systems three or four times a year. Nurses on the floor complained with some justification that the typical doctor was much more likely to repeatedly ask the same question about the location of one or another piece of equipment (or ask someone to fetch it) than to invest time in learning where things were. Working on their own time, three staff nurses prepared an orientation booklet for the new residents. It included a floor plan of the unit and detailed information about the location of equipment and supplies. Apart from its purely information value, the hand-out was meant to convey a subtle message to the doctors—that they should make an effort to find things themselves rather than to continually ask harried nurses.

The monthly orientation meeting was planned to include a walkthrough of the "welcome to Barnard 5" orientation booklet and additional information aimed at acquainting new residents with the unit. For example, they would be warned not to leave hypodermic needles lying about but to use proper means of disposal and to return charts to their proper slots in the chart rack after being used. The three-person orientation committee worked up a list of RNs who would be responsible for leading the orientation meetings on a rotating basis.

The first orientation meeting was scheduled for January 15, 1977. The nursing staff contributed out-of-pocket monies to provide coffee and doughnuts for the occasion. A nurse who had little previous involvement in the project ran the orientation. Four other Barnard 5 staff members were present, including Bruce Gould. Three sleepy-eyed but sympathetic members of the house staff sat through the presentation, asked a few routine questions, thanked the staff, and left. The Barnard 5 group considered the meeting a major success.

Thereafter orientation sessions ranging from fifteen minutes to a half an hour were held on or around the first of every month. The doctors were under no official pressure to attend the sessions, and the Barnard staff soon discovered that the success or failure of the monthly doctors' meeting depended on how much cooperation they got from the chief resident. Some chief residents were eager to cooperate. But other months the experience was a disheartening one for the staff as the following example, taken from the notes of a research team member, illustrates.

> Early in the morning of March 1, 1977, Bruce Gould approached the chief resident, Dr. Arkin, to make sure that the residents' orientation, scheduled for the period following morning rounds, would proceed as planned. Dr. Arkin assured Gould that the residents would be there. After rounds were completed, however, Arkin sent four residents off the floor to observe an operation, leaving a single new resident and five disappointed nursing staff members sitting amid untouched trays of coffee, doughnuts, bagels, and cream cheese. Angrily, the group delegated Cathy Thomas to go to Dr. Saltzman and explain what happened. She did. At three o'clock that afternoon, all the residents except Dr. Arkin were reassembled in the nurses' lounge on Barnard 5 and, the orientation proceeded.

Despite the hit-or-miss nature of the residents' orientations, Barnard 5 staff members saw them as one of the major accomplishments of the quality of work life project.

Staff Conferences

The second action step was to revive the staff meetings initiated by the NQWC representative and continued by Eric Moore under the deceptively concrete name of the Barnard 5 Task Force.

Steve Meyer believed that a representative group, as the task force was intended to be, was impractical; it was too difficult to arrange meetings for employees working on three separate shifts, and the format tended to limit the composition of the group to a small core of regular participants. Instead, Meyer proposed shift-based staff conferences. He felt that weekly meetings among work group members along with occasional cross-shift meetings would be a more effective vehicle for improving the communications flow on the unit. Moreover, the staff conference model followed existing lines of authority on the unit. Since the consultants' diagnostic work revealed a great deal of confusion about role responsibilities, particularly in the relationship between the clinical supervisor and the senior clinical nurse, the staff meetings would allow opportunities for needed role clarification.

Staff conferences began on the day shift. The leadership of the meetings alternated between the senior clinical nurse, Cathy Thomas, and clinical supervisor, Ivan Edwards. When both were absent, a staff nurse would take the leadership role. Steve Meyer attended most of the early meetings of the project and assumed the role of facilitator. On several occasions, Meyer attempted to clarify the implications of decisions made by the group, such as who was responsible for what tasks and who should be contacted. Meyer tried to make sure that staff members followed through on decisions made in previous meetings. He also acted as a channel of communication between Marullo and staff on the unit. In short, Meyer did what a consultant in his situation is supposed to do, and the group saw him as supportive and helpful.

Overall, the consultants viewed the staff conferences as a means of improving the capacity of Barnard 5 staff members to work together as a group. The content of the meetings varied, although relatively little time was spent on designated QWL project activities such as reports of steering committee meetings and the residents' orientation. The bulk of the meeting time was devoted to routine matters of nursing care—briefings on new procedures, introducing new reporting forms, administrative announcements, and occasional clinical discussions of specific patients. The idea of scheduling a weekly meeting for all levels of staff on a nursing unit is hardly a novel idea, even in so traditional a hospital as Parkside. But the staff meetings made a difference in the quality of working life on the unit, and perhaps as important, they provided an incentive for suggesting other, more far-reaching types of innovations.

Having established a certain success on Barnard 5, the Evans team began to take a broader look at the Parkside system as they renewed their search for a more powerful constituency. Evans and Meyer established a closer relationship with Dr. Saltzman, the respected surgeon on the steering committee who was to remain an active participant throughout the life of the project. With Saltzman's backing, Evans presented an overview of the project at surgical grand rounds and got an attentive although rather polite reception. Evans and Meyer also continued to work with Nancy Marullo to improve nursing management in Barnard Pavilion. Still, the Evans group did not have the backing of a senior manager within the diffuse Parkside system, and without such support, it was unlikely that any unit-level reforms would continue beyond the limited tenure of the consultant group.

With this in mind, Evans asked for and received a place on the agenda of the January 24, 1977 monthly meeting of Parkside's Senior Management Group. The Evans team made extensive preparations for the meeting. They wrote a long progress report and had it distributed to members of the senior management group, or SMG, prior to the meeting. They enlisted Bruce Gould and Dr. Saltzman to come and present their perspectives as participants in the Barnard 5 project.

Steve Meyer found out after the meeting that Harvey Hertz, the hospital director, had no idea that the QWL project would be discussed at the meeting. This accounted for his look of surprise when the consultants, the two Barnard 5 representatives, and a member of the Columbia research team entered the hospital's main conference room at the alloted agenda point about halfway through the meeting. Along with the seven members of the SMG there were about a dozen department chiefs at the meeting. Meredith Klein introduced the consultants, Gould, and Saltzman to the group and quickly turned the floor over to Gould, who delivered a spirited, if somewhat disjointed, presentation on the impact of the project on Barnard 5. Then Steve Meyer called upon Dr. Saltzman who gave an equally positive statement on the project. Saltzman remarked that:

> There's been a dramatic change in the involvement of people on the floor since Evans took over. I've seen a real improvement in communication between the doctors and nurses. And morale is much better now.

The audience appeared sympathetic, but there were few comments after Bill Evans closed the presentation. Finally, the chief of the ambulatory care department expressed a critical opinion about tangible results, such as quantified improvements in patient care. A few of the department heads came to the project's defense by pointing out that morale change, while intangible, is real and significant. This could have provided a strategic opening to discuss the ultimate goals of the project and to build a constituency for it, but the time allotted to the consultants had run out.

Throughout the presentation and the ensuing discussion, the hospital director said nothing. But he did provide some closing comments. His tone was positive but distant—reminiscent of his comments during the first and only QWL project meeting he had attended, back in August of 1975. The project, in his words, "was essential . . . because we need to know if we can do this kind of constituency building in this environment." He closed by saying that "The management group should take a closer look at the project—but not right now." Immediately Meyer suggested that the consultants meet with the management team at some point in March or April. The director responded by saying simply that the consultants would get a place on the agenda if they requested it in time.

Following the meeting Evans, Meyer, and Hartman got together for a short debriefing and planning session. They were manifestly disappointed with the meeting and angry about the lukewarm reception they got from the director. They were also angry at Meredith Klein for not providing any real support during the meeting or even telling the director that the group would be making a presentation. Meyer remarked that he wanted to go to the funding agency at HEW and tell them that the only way the project would work would be to have it redesignated as a management project. The director was not going to take it seriously until he had more of a sense of ownership. Evans talked Meyer out of the idea, but the team resolved that it was impossible to continue without a greater measure of legitimacy. The consultants had gained credibility on Barnard 5, the staff conferences were going well, and the orientation sessions for new residents were being held on a regular basis; but other, more elaborate intervention plans required support from the larger system.

Two weeks after their meeting with the senior management group, the consultants met for a day-long strategy meeting. They reached two important conclusions: First, the steering committee must be confronted and asked to provide a much greater degree of support for the project. Second, in its present form, the steering committee was extremely ineffective; it was unwieldy and included too many people with little power. Echoing his earlier statement, Meyer asserted that the project had to get closer to the management of the hospital if it was going to win any real support. With this in mind, he proposed a smaller, more influential subcommittee within the overall project steering committee. The subcommittee would include the director of nursing and at least one other member of the senior management group (Dr. Mauer, the head of the clinical services division, had already expressed an interest in becoming involved in the project), a representative from the Hospital Workers' Union, one from the Parkside chapter of the State Nurses' Association, and a physician, presumably Dr. Saltzman. Meyer believed that a smaller group would be able to meet more often, respond to events more quickly, and, because of its membership, would have a better chance of securing attention from Parkside management. A smaller, more cohesive group would also encourage its members to exercise their formal authority in the service of QWL project activities. In short, the consultants wanted an executive subcommittee that would be the union-management policy-making body called for in the quality of work life model. This is also what Moe Kurtzman was seeking. On several occasions, Kurtzman complained that the committee had become top-heavy with management personnel and that if it was going to be a viable, decision-making group, it would have to be restructured so that each of the constituent groups would be represented by one person. Meyer's plan was virtually identical to what Kurtzman was asking for, although the underlying rationale was different; from the consultant's perspective, the essential question was how to increase the level of commitment from both the Hospital Workers' Union and management.

The next day, Evans and Meyer presented the restructuring proposal to the steering committee. Evans told the group that despite the progress on Barnard 5, the project wasn't going to get very far without involvement from both top management and the unions. Management wasn't interested now and probably would not take the project seriously unless it had more control. The proposed subcommittee might provide the key for capturing management's attention. Evans asserted that a smaller group would also address Moe Kurtzman's longstanding complaint that the committee was no longer a core union-management group. Almost as an afterthought, Evans offered words of reassurance to the full committee: it would *still* be the project steering committee; whatever proposals the subcommittee came up with would be reviewed by the larger group.

The immediate reaction to Evans' proposal was silence. Then, one by one, committee members raised their objections to the idea of restructuring the committee. Blanche Reiner said that no action could be taken without the approval of the Hospital Workers' Union, and since Moe Kurtzman was not at the meeting, she would not vote for the consultants' plan. (Reiner apparently did not hear or chose not to acknowledge a point Meyer made earlier in the meeting—that Kurtzman did not intend to end his boycott of steering committee meetings *until* a smaller working committee was formed.) Others responded more directly. An irate Gertrude Thayer said: "There should be no subcommittees unless there are specific objectives. Preserve this committee and make it work. I will not stand by and see the emasculation of this committee."

Steve Meyer responded angrily: "What we are talking about is the emasculation of the project. I have serious doubts that without a major change, we will be able to continue."

More heated discussion followed. One participant made a passing reference to the consultants' "divide and conquer strategy." Evans and Meyer saw that they were getting nowhere and backed off. Meyer closed by saying that he and Evans would try to continue within the present framework but that they would probably raise the subcommittee issue again in a few months if there was no significant change in the project's status within the hospital. For the time being, a major component of the Evans group's emerging strategy had failed to win necessary approval.

The Barnard 5 Staffing Crisis

The consultants' problems did not end with the steering committee, the union, and the management. Staffing had long been a major point of conflict in Barnard Pavilion. Now there were serious threats to the encouraging but still fragile developments on Barnard 5. Prior to the selection of Barnard 5 as the experimental site for the quality of work life project, the State Nurses' Association had filed a grievance charging that understaffing within the pavilion was threatening patient care and creating intolerable working conditions for RNs. Parkside's management responded by hiring a consulting firm, Healthtech, to carry out a patient classification survey. The study's major objective was to quantify the amount of nursing care provided to patients on all nursing units within Parkside and to use these data in conjunction with established nursing care standards to set recommended staffing levels throughout the hospital.

Regardless of its intended purpose, the Healthtech survey created substantial anxiety among employees at all levels. The Hospital Workers' Union feared that survey results would provide a rationale for layoffs. Many nurses believed that the Healthtech standards did not accurately reflect the scope and magnitude of nurses' duties, and that the study would ultimately recommend fewer, not more, staff. Unit level supervisors felt that the survey was insensitive to important differences between units. For example, the clinical supervisor for Barnard 8, a specialized surgery unit, noted that there were only 19 beds on the unit and that by overall standards the ratio of nursing staff to patients was quite high. But due to the nature of medical problems on the unit, nurses were required to do an inordinate amount of patient teaching. Her concern was that the patient classification survey would not give adequate consideration to extraordinary teaching needs in the setting of recommended staffing levels.

As the chief nursing department administrator in Barnard Pavilion, Nancy Marullo was in a position to separate fact from fantasy and to assure unit members and her own supervisory staff that the Healthtech survey was a necessary step in setting up a rational staffing system that would benefit both employees and patients. Instead, her actions tended to make things worse. For example, she refused to acknowledge the legitimacy of the clinical supervisors' fear that the patient classification project would produce both winners and losers. She made unsubstantiated promises to pavilion staff that new nurses would be hired by a certain date; when the date passed and no additional staff were forthcoming, she lost a substantial measure of credibility and trust.

Worries about the Healthtech survey and dissatisfaction with present staffing levels were as strong on Barnard 5 as anywhere else in the Hospital. Forced weekend duty on short notice, unscheduled overtime, and widespread confusion over nursing coverage were the rule. During one of the staff conferences, one nursing aide told of being reprimanded for not showing up for work on the previous Monday and for not calling in; in fact, she had no idea that she had been rescheduled to work that day. The worsening staff situation on the floor threatened to unravel whatever gains had been made by Meyer's team-building efforts. On several occasions, staff members told Meyer directly that they were not going to invest any time in QWL project activities until some resolution to the staffing crisis was found.

Evans and Meyer made the bold decision to turn the staffing and scheduling mess into a major focal point of project activity. With their encouragement, staff conferences were turned into brainstorming sessions aimed at coming up with possible solutions. Evans, acting as an intermediary between Barnard 5 staff and Marullo, obtained Marullo's commitment that if staff could come up with a plan that would give everyone a scheduled weekend off every other week while still satisfying minimum staff requirements, she would seriously consider the plan for adoption. In effect, the bargain struck between Marullo and unit staff became a major test of the validity of the quality of work life concept.

A three-person committee, headed by day shift RN Ellen Mackey, volunteered to draft a scheduling plan. They spent several weeks on the project and spent a considerable amount of their own time on it. Finally, they were satisfied that they had put together a workable scheme. They presented their work to the day shift staff conference, and it was greeted enthusiastically. Then the group went to Marullo, who rejected the plan almost immediately but offered to meet with the staff and present her rationale.

The meeting was one of the best attended and most intense staff conferences since the Evans group took over as project consultants. Eleven staff members were present—the entire complement from the day and evening shifts—along with Evans, Edwards, and Marullo.

Marullo led off by speaking directly to the issue of the impracticality of the scheduling plan. She contended that it set unconscionably low staffing levels for weekend tours of duty, specifically a "two and one" (two RNs and one nursing aide) arrangement on the weekend day shift. It also would have meant minimal staff coverage on the evening and night shifts throughout the week. Marullo not only condemned the plan, she openly questioned the nurses' commitment to patient care. Turning to Ellen Mackey, she remarked: "I want to ask you how you feel about shortchanging your patients. How does it affect your image of yourself as a professional?"

Later on, Marullo softened her position. She was not rejecting the plan, she said, but merely stating the facts; it could never work given present staffing levels. However, the early Healthtech survey results indicated that Barnard 5 should be staffed to provide 4.6 nursing hours per patient per day. Since the unit's present staffing was far below this standard, one should expect to see new nurses on the floor within a matter of three or four months. At that point, the group's staffing proposal might be realistic.

By the end of the meeting, there had been a great deal of frank discussion about the problems facing the floor. Marullo listened carefully, made some suggestions, and regained some credibility. But no one believed her prediction that the coming months would bring a resolution to the staffing crisis. Indeed, there were strong rumors of impending layoffs amid reports that the budget deficit for the year would be large. Marullo herself made a passing reference to the possibility of layoffs.

As the scheduling plan disappeared, so did the consultants' immediate hopes for expanding the scope of project activity on Barnard 5. The fiasco confirmed the consultants' belief that little of significance could be accomplished without higher level management support. But how to win this support was by no means clear.

INTERPRETIVE SUMMARY

When the Evans team took over as consultants to the project, there was an implicit directive to show some demonstrable success on the pilot unit, Barnard 5. The Evans group soon discovered that a single nursing unit has little autonomy within the larger hospital system, and that it would be futile to make a major effort to improve the performance and quality of work life of Barnard 5 while leaving the larger system of the hospital unchanged. Systemic change meant bringing management into the picture—hence the consultants began to work with Nancy Marullo, the assistant director of nursing, who was the top manager in the pavilion. But apart from the problems that were inherent in Marullo's personal style—her inclination to move "in all sorts of directions as once"—she lacked the authority of managers at her level in other types of organizations. The consultants were discovering just how complicated a large hospital is and how difficult it can be to find a handle for change. Evans and his colleagues then tried to improve their position by attempting to win the support of the senior management of the hospital and by getting some lasting commitment from the leader of the Hospital Workers' Union at Parkside. Neither initiative appeared to be successful, at least immediately. The consultants began to see the hospital—accurately—as a highly political organization. They realized that they would not get very far without doing a fair amount of political base building themselves. But in hindsight, it seems apparent that the consultants' energy was being absorbed by the need to assume a political role, and that this detracted seriously from their efforts to implement the program of change described in their ambitious organizational development plan.

CHAPTER SEVEN

Building Ownership
The Evolution of the Consultants' Strategy

In the aftermath of the scheduling conflict, Evans and Meyer tried to keep the lines of communication between Marullo and her staff as open as possible. At the same time, they began to consider the possibility of transferring the project to a different part of the hospital. They were looking for an assistant director of nursing who would provide more enthusiasm for the project than Marullo did and who enjoyed a close, trusting working relationship with her staff. Locating such a person among the half dozen other assistant directors would not be easy; the consultants still had few contacts within the hospital, and they were hardly in a position to make a public recruiting effort. So while they continued their search for a suitable client, they doubled their efforts to improve the nursing management hierarchy within Barnard Pavilion.

The consultants learned from Marullo that the nursing department was undergoing a major reorganization. A new supervisory position was being created, that of unit manager. The unit manager would be responsible for much of the administrative load currently handled by staff RNs. The reorganization plan also called for upgrading the job description of unit clerk and reviewing all other nursing staff job descriptions up to the level of assistant director. Evans and Meyer saw the reorganization as an opportunity to connect the QWL project to an important organizational change. It was no secret that the nursing department needed a major overhaul. Poor organization, unclear reporting relationships, low staff morale, and high turnover among entry level nurses plagued the department and compromised attempts to improve patient care. If Evans was able to pull off a successful intervention, it would gain much needed credibility for the quality of work life project.

With this in mind, Evans went to Marullo and asked if he and Meyer could play a role in the implementation of the reorganization plan. Evans told her that the consultants could help to clarify the process of change—whom to bring together to solve problems and how to insure that tasks are followed through to completion. Marullo seemed hesitant, but suggested that the consultants might get involved by reorganizing the nursing station on Barnard 5 and helping to revive the concept of team nursing on the floor. Evans saw these as peripheral, unimportant tasks. He countered by telling Marullo that it made better sense to attempt reforms on a pavilionwide basis—not within the limited arena of a single nursing floor. Marullo did not reject Evans' idea, but she reacted strongly when Meyer suggested that the project steering committee be given a briefing on possible links between the QWL project and nursing changes within Barnard Pavilion. She flatly rejected steering committee involvement on the grounds that nursing care reform was a sole prerogative of the department of nursing. She also denied that the considerable time that Evans and Meyer spent with her and her subordinates had anything to do with the QWL project. Meyer tried another tactic by asking Marullo if he and Evans could participate in a scheduled in-service training program for senior clinical nurses and clinical supervisors, the two principal middle management positions in the nursing department. Again, Marullo said no; the consultants should limit themselves to the newly spawned team nursing project on Barnard 5.

In short, Marullo made it very clear that the QWL project would remain marginal to the major organizational changes taking place within Barnard Pavilion and within the nursing division as a whole. Evans and Meyer were discovering that Marullo's position reflected that of Meredith Klein, the director of nursing. Not only did Klein fail to bring Evans and Meyer into the planning process of the divisional reorganization, she seemed unwilling to commit substantial resources to QWL project activities. Her only indication of further support was in reference to a project that was being set up by Dr. Mauer, the director of clinical services, and the third member of the consulting team, Dan Hartman. In response to a question from Evans, Klein confided that the QWL project lacked essential support within the hospital's senior management group. She and the clinical services director were for it, but the real issue was Harvey Hertz, the hospital director, who had little interest in supporting a joint union-management change project. The hospital faced an enormous deficit and growing uncertainties over future reimbursement levels from third party insurers such as Medicare. These problems had important ramifications for labor relations within the hospital. Parkside needed additional nursing staff—the early results from the Healthtech survey confirmed this—but the deficit precluded any new hiring for at least six months. And even then, monies going to increase the ranks of general duty RNs would have to come from staff reductions in other areas. In all likelihood, this would mean laying off nonprofessional employees. The Hospital Workers' Union knew this, and shortly after Evans' talk with Klein, a large group of union delegates staged a sit-in in the office of the special assistant to the director in protest of rumored lay-off plans. Given this turbulent environment, Klein said, "Hertz does not want to involve the union in management decisions." As if to emphasize the marginality of the quality of work life project, Klein ended by informing Evans that she would no longer have the time to attend steering committee meetings on a regular basis.

Their meeting with Klein deepened the consultants' pessimism. It was now March of 1977, seven months since the Evans team was chosen to resurrect the project. Their frustration with the steering committee and with Marullo left them wondering if it would ever be possible to establish a viable consultant-client relationship within the hospital. The alternatives were limited. Meyer's earlier proposal—to go to HEW to try to have the project redesignated as a management-sponsored change effort—was never raised again, perhaps because the consultants knew that it was unlikely that the funding source would agree to it. Another option was to acknowledge the extreme difficulties inherent in a union-management project within a hostile labor relations setting and pull out. Despite their pessimism, this was never given serious consideration, at least in the presence of the research team. The third option was to continue on their course and to keep searching for a sympathetic authority figure in the hospital. In the end, this is what the consultants chose to do.

THE CLINICAL SERVICES PROJECT

In mid-March, the search for a QWL supporter from management finally paid off. Dan Hartman, the third member of the Evans team, who had been working more or less independently of Evans and Meyer, made contact with Dr. Jack Mauer, the new director of the Clinical Services Division of Parkside. Mauer, who had a Ph.D. in hospital administration, had come to Parkside from a similar position in a smaller hospital in the midwest. Mauer was enthusiastic, hardworking, and committed to change. And there was certainly a need for change within the clinical services division. Administratively, the division included twenty specialized medical departments including radiology, nuclear medicine, respiratory therapy, the blood bank, and several laboratory based departments including microbiology and chemistry. The division also encompassed the library of the hospital and medical school. Most of the clinical services departments were headed by physicians, and though many had international reputations within their medical specialities, few were competent administrators. One of Mauer's first major reforms was a complete reorganization of the radiology department, one of the largest of the clinical services, and, by reputation, among the worst managed. But Mauer also wanted to take on the problem of lack of coordination between the clinical departments—each functioned as an autonomous "fiefdom" of its physician director—and the lack of coordination between departments and nursing units.

Mauer was intent on bringing rational management to the division. He took immediate steps to improve the weak management information systems of each of the clinical departments, and he devoted considerable attention to the design and implementation of quantitative performance measures. But, by training and temperament, he was also aware of the people side of management reform. And he was a strong believer in research. Thus he was receptive to Hartman's invitation to become involved in the quality of work life project. Within a couple of weeks after he was approached, Mauer committed himself, his staff, and the division to a major organizational change effort within the QWL framework.

There were two basic parts to the Hartman-Mauer plan. The first was a large-scale survey feedback project. A survey questionnaire covering employee opinions on several areas of organizational and work group performance would be administered to all division employees. The resulting data would be collated and given back to department directors and employee groups and used to identify specific change objectives. Task forces comprised of different levels of employees would implement these changes. Then employees would be resurveyed. The second wave of data would indicate how well the initial change objectives were met and would provide the empirical base for the next feedback cycle. The plan followed the basic survey feedback change strategy. (See Bowers & Franklin, 1976; Nadler, 1977.)

The second part of the plan was an "organizational mirroring" project (see French & Bell, 1978) that would involve staff members from several clinical departments and nursing units. Data would be gathered on how employees in a department or nursing floor are perceived by their counterparts with whom they interact. For example, blood bank staff members would receive feedback data from nursing unit employees—feedback that would include perceptions of problems (for example, blood arriving late on the floor) and examples of superior performance. In turn, blood bank staff would offer feedback to nursing unit employees. The objective of the exercise was to enable a department or unit to see how its performance was viewed by others—hence the mirroring element of the plan. The next step would be to hold joint meetings between departments and nursing floors to work on problems identified in the mirroring data.

Evans and Meyer greeted Hartman's plan with ambivalence. They were excited about the prospect of a committed and powerful client in the person of Mauer, but they weren't pleased with the fact that Hartman had made an essentially unilateral decision to commit the consultant team to a plan that appeared to have little relationship to the Barnard-based core activities of the quality of work life project. The "Mauer Project," as it was labelled, was a fait accompli. It involved a sudden shift in the attention and resources of the team at a point when the fixed, depleted consultant budget was a salient issue in the team's forward planning discussions.

The origins of the Mauer project also reflected a difference in the style and philosophy of the consultants. Hartman had little commitment to the bottom-up ideology that suffused the QWL project. He viewed his role as that of a management consultant who had searched for and found a willing, capable manager to consult for. Once he reached an agreement with Mauer, he moved rapidly, unfettered by any obligation to brief the unions or weigh the opinions of lower level employees. In contrast, while Evans and Meyer had serious misgivings about the participative, union-management change model, they accepted the slow and often frustrating process of constituency building as part of their contract.

The most difficult immediate problem facing Evans was how to "sell" the steering committee on a project that had never been presented or discussed before. This would not be easy in the context of the residue of ill feelings left by the restructuring fiasco.

The clinical services project was the major agenda item of the thirty-sixth steering committee meeting, which was held on March 29, 1977. Present were Sally McBride of the State Nurses' Association; Loretta Musial of the hospital's training and development staff; Blanche Reiner and an assistant from social services; George Brown, an assistant personnel manager who was representing hospital management;

Nancy Marullo; Dr. Saltzman; Dr. Mauer, the director of clinical services; the three members of the consultant team; and two observers
from Columbia. Mauer started the meeting with an extended presentation covering the project's objectives and time frame. Dan Hartman
added some comments on the importance of the project. The reaction
from the steering committee was mixed. George Brown asked
Hartman several challenging questions while making the point that
this would be only the latest of a long series of organizational change
projects in the clinical services division—none of which had produced
any lasting change. Hartman retorted that *this* project was different;
the employees would have ownership, and this would help make it
work. Blanche Reiner offered some favorable comments, but she questioned the apparent lack of Hospital Workers' Union involvement and
wondered aloud if the union was still part of the quality of work life
project. Loretta Musial and Evans assured her that HWU was still in;
it was an unavoidable crisis that had kept Moe Kurtzman from attending the meeting. Still Reiner wondered, "Where are the workers in
all this?" Evans answered that the survey would elicit the feelings and
opinions of staff members at *all* levels. Hartman was less accommoda-
tive; turning to Reiner, he said sharply: "I wouldn't have been able to
get my foot in the door if I didn't start from the top." He then called for
a steering committee endorsement of the clincal services plan since it
was intended to further one of the principal goals of the quality of work
life project—better patient care. Reiner countered: "Better patient
care. You're asking for an endorsement of motherhood."

But in the end, the consultants got the approval of the steering
committee. Evans brought things to a close by setting up a meeting
with Saltzman, Marullo, Hartman, and himself to begin to coordinate
the new project with ongoing QWL activities in Barnard Pavilion.

BRINGING THE HOSPITAL WORKERS' UNION BACK IN

HWU's participation in the QWL project remained marginal throughout the spring of 1977. Moe Kurtzman had not been to a steering
committee meeting in several months, and while his absence was usually ignored, someone would occasionally raise the question of the legitimacy of an expensive, time-consuming, and ostensibly union-
management project in which the principal union was nowhere in
evidence.

Kurtzman had his share of problems. Rumors of impending layoffs
made his official presence on a joint union-management committee a

delicate issue within union ranks. He was embroiled in what seemed to be a continuous series of conflicts over supervision, work load, and the job security of his membership. He told the Columbia research team that labor relations had never been as bad as they were at this point. Moreover, a worsening physical disability reduced his ability to move about the hospital and stay in touch with his constituency. He felt isolated and surrounded by hostile forces.

Bill Evans made a special effort to maintain contact with Kurtzman. Throughout this period, their personal relationship was the only real connection between the union and the quality of work life project. Evans listened to Kurtzman tell of his conflicts with nursing and the hospital administration and how the management had moved him to a smaller, less accessible office without a telephone. But the price he set on rejoining the steering committee—a basic restructuring and the reduction of management representation—was still unacceptable.

So Evans and Meyer began to work on another strategy to win union support. The lack of HWU participation in the Barnard 5 project was becoming a matter of public concern. The project officer from HEW qualified his favorable assessment of the Evans team in a recent site visit by commenting on the apparent lack of HWU members in visible project roles. Bruce Gould and other active RNs on Barnard 5 continued to reach out to nursing aides and assistants and housekeeping staff without much success. Kurtzman was aware of these perceptions and commented to Evans that the low status workers in the hospital think about working conditions and patient care a great deal more than is recognized; the real problem is that most do not feel confident in speaking out in public.

Kurtzman's comment led Evans to schedule a meeting with union delegates and HWU members on Barnard 5. He learned that the delegates were also concerned about improving the communications abilities of the membership. With this in mind, Evans proposed a training program in interpersonal skill building for nursing aides and assistants, unit clerks, and other nonsupervisory staff. It would include training in conflict resolution, listening, how to run an effective meeting, problem solving, and how to communicate ideas more forcefully and constructively. Evans emphasized that a "packaged program" would not work; the shape and content of the program would have to address the express needs of HWU members.

Evans and Meyer also spent a great deal of time meeting individually with members of the steering committee to get input on the proposed training program. Blanche Reiner suggested the need for a training session on employees' feelings about death and dying. Doctors and nurses receive training on coping with death in their professional education, but the person who cleans the floor, who also has contact with dying patients, has to bear it alone. Reiner believed that the high rate of turnover and sick time among nonprofessional employees was connected to the lack of opportunities for dealing with the anxiety and depression caused by the immediacy of death in their place of work. She accepted readily Evans' suggestion that she run a training session on the topic.

As Evans had intended, planning for the training program helped to weave the hospital workers back into the fabric of the QWL project. Kurtzman was now fully committed to working with the consultants even though the problems with the steering committee had not been solved. But the evolution of the training program also illustrated the slow, labored pace of the QWL project and the inherent difficulties of a bottom-up approach to organizational change. Eight months elapsed between the first announcement of the training program in March of 1977 and the first training session in December. By that point, as will be seen, much of the employee optimism toward the QWL project had disappeared, and the potential contribution of the training program toward building union and worker involvement had been reduced considerably.

Moe Kurtzman returned to the steering committee in May of 1977. By then, the consultants' stance toward the group had changed. They abandoned their efforts to work with the steering committee as a whole and instead sought closer collaboration with individual committee members with authority in the hospital. They concluded that the steering committee would never be an effective decision-making body and that the joint union-management project model was not a viable one, at least in the context of Parkside. In effect, the client of Evans and his colleagues was not a single entity but a disparate set of interest groups within the hospital—the staff on Barnard 5, Nancy Marullo and her subordinates, Meredith Klein, and Robert Mauer, as well as the hospital workers. Each of these contituencies was the focus of a separate change project with few direct connections between them.

Since the "hub of the wheel" metaphor no longer described the steering committee, its structure was hardly a matter of importance anymore. So when Moe Kurtzman presented his restructuring proposal to the group on May 6, it was basically anticlimatic. This didn't stop Kurtzman from making a rousing presentation. He praised Evans and Meyer and said:

> Things have really turned around. I'm getting good feedback from my people. It's the first time in two years since this thing began that they are positive about it. Even my skeptical delegates are for it now.

Going on to his major point, he argued that the steering committee must be scaled down and that members of the Barnard 5 Task Force should be allowed to attend only when invited. It was a measure of his distance from the actual workings of the project that he did not know that the task force had been dropped shortly after the Evans team had taken over the consultant role. Nancy Marullo's curt reply to Kurtzman's proposal was:

> It basically doesn't matter. They (the Barnard 5 staff) don't want to come anyway. It's a hassle for them. Bruce Gould may still want to come, but Ivan Edwards certainly doesn't care.

Marullo later commented that: "The whole project is at a standstill—it has to be revitalized." A moment later she complimented Steve Meyer for the excellent work he was doing with her administrative staff. In Marullo's mind, there was no paradox here; the QWL project was thoroughly separate from (and marginal to) her own administrative reform and the consultants' involvement in the reform process.

A month later, on June 7, the steering committee met to hear the Evans team's briefing on the status of the QWL project at the halfway point in the consultants' eighteen-month contract. As usual, Evans gave an upbeat assessment. The clinical services feedback project and the organization mirroring project were "up and running." The Barnard 5 staff conferences and doctors' orientation were going well. Ivan Edwards added some positive comments to Evans' overview. There were no decisions to be made, and the Evans team asked the committee for nothing. In the consultants' overall strategy, the steering committee had ceased to be the center of the quality of work life project.

Indeed, the steering committee met only two more times—in October 1977 and at the time of the project's termination in July of 1978. At the October meeting, the consultants finally won approval for the proposed steering committee working group, consisting of Meredith Klein, Robert Mauer, Nancy Marullo, and Moe Kurtzman. The steering committee decided that the smaller group would meet on a biweekly basis and would provide the much needed vehicle for acting quickly on urgent project-related matters.

This working group met three times during late October and early November of 1977. Each time the sole agenda item was selecting participants for the upcoming Barnard 5 training program. By the end of the series of meetings it was no longer a program for HWU members exclusively, nor was it limited to Barnard 5. A housekeeping supervisor whose responsibilities included all of Barnard Pavilion was added along with an evening nursing supervisor, a unit clerk from Barnard

4, and a few others. Basically, there were not enough HWU-affiliated staff members who volunteered to attend the sessions to make it worthwhile as an exclusively union effort, and there were a number of non-HWU personnel who were interested in attending. There was little debate over the revised composition of the training group.

The steering committee working group then decided to hold off on meeting again until after the first training session on December 7. As it turned out, the group did not meet until the final month of the project, June of 1978.

Thus, over the final eight months of the Parkside Quality of Work Life Project, the core union-management group no longer functioned. Instead, there were a number of basically autonomous subprojects that commanded the attention of the Evans team. In the following chapter, the course of each of these projects will be described.

INTERPRETIVE SUMMARY

In discussing the wayward course of the Parkside Quality of Work Life Project up to this point, it is worth considering what the project might have accomplished if conditions had been more favorable and if some of what had been learned over the years about the design of QWL projects had been applied at Parkside. QWL consultants now give a great deal of emphasis to training the key participants in the types of interpersonal and group skills encompassed by the Barnard training program. To be effective, however, training activities should be carried out *before* the initiation of QWL interventions. If successfully implemented, preproject training yields several benefits. Participants learn what is expected of them, how to work together effectively, and how to deal with conflict.

One can imagine that with successful start-up training and a more supportive management and union leadership, the evolution of the Barnard 5 pilot unit project might have gone as follows: The staff of the unit and the consultants would work together to identify various means of improving quality of work life and patient care. The project steering committee would review the unit group's work. Unrealistic suggestions, such as the scheduling plan, would still be rejected, but the reasons for the rejection would be made clear. Steering committee members would provide the assistance necessary to implement worthwhile proposals that go beyond the boundaries of the nursing unit. For example, with Dr. Saltzman's support, Barnard 5 staff might have been given the opportunity to meet with the physician in charge of residency training in order to work out arrangements for scheduling orientation sessions for residents throughout the hospital. Bruce Gould and his collaborators on the orientation booklet would be given time to function as "consultants" to staff on other floors. A similar arrangement would be made for diffusing the staff conference model throughout the department of nursing. During the implementation, the unions would take an active role—to make sure that changes in work procedures do not violate contract provisions, but also to help employees to articulate their own interests in organizational change. The needle issue, for example, might have become a special project concern and the focus of a joint task force of HWU members and supervisors who would work out new procedures for disposing of contaminated syringes and who would monitor the results.

Clearly, this in not the way the project evolved. But many of the conditions that are necessary for a sucessful project *were* present. It is important to identify these positive forces for change and the impediments to change that eventually won out.

The consultants were notably successful in reviving the project on Barnard 5. It was not an easy task. The first meetings that Steve Meyer scheduled on the floor were lifeless affairs. Staff members remained disillusioned from the Wheaton failure, the scheduling conflict with the assistant director of nursing, and the constant pressures of understaffing. But gradually, the project began to pick up speed. Joining the core group of three or four RNs that kept the project alive during slow periods were several other RNs—some of whom were new to the floor and unaffected by the Wheaton debacle—and others who had taken a wait-and-see position. Perhaps more significantly, several nonprofessional employees—unit clerks, nursing assistants, and housekeepers—began to participate in the QWL staff conferences on the floor. Even the unit clerk on the day shift, who had come to symbolize staff resistance to the project, began to attend and participate in the weekly conferences.

These meetings provided a sanctioned escape from the normally authoritarian system of work relations on the unit. For the nonprofessionals, the meetings were a change from their usually passive roles as followers of orders from physicians, staff nurses, and supervisors. For the nurses, the conferences provided an opportunity to look beyond immediate work problems and explore ways to provide greater freedom and opportunities for personal and professional development. Apart from being a supportive forum for the airing of feelings about work and coworkers and for testing new ideas, the staff meetings also increased the flow of patient care information among the unit's employees. Over a period of several months, the character of the staff conferences changed from that of short, quasi-military briefings run by the senior clinical nurse to expansive, vibrant meetings that often ran far beyond their alloted time. It was not uncommon to see staff members in "civilian" clothes who had come in on a day off to attend a meeting and to report on the activities of one of the ad hoc working groups that had emerged to handle specific projects. Nonprofessional employees who had always taken a back seat—in a literal sense—throughout the course of the meetings began to sit interspersed with the RNs and, on occasion, a surgical resident. The QWL staff conferences and the support work that went into them gave real meaning to the concept of the patient care team.

An excerpt from the observation notes of a member of the Columbia research team illustrates the content of these meetings.

> Cathy Thomas brought up a change in the NPO procedures. Up to now, RNs were responsible for collecting all information about restriction on patients' diets and for sending this information at the appropriate time to the dietary department. The new regulation gives the responsibility to the unit clerk and puts an 11:30 AM deadline on all next-day dietary changes.
>
> Karen Sullivan, a day shift unit clerk, began to complain about 'another thing being dumped on the unit clerk.' She looked over to the evening shift unit clerk for support. Responding to her anger, Cathy Thomas told her that the unit clerks were not being singled out for more work; RNs were also being stuck with a whole new set of paperwork responsibilities. Then, Cathy and another RN suggested the idea of a summary sheet that could be used to record dietary information from the patient cards that were kept by the RNs. The summary sheet would eliminate the need for the clerk to run around to every patient's bed to check the bedside record of diet orders. Nurses, Cathy suggested, should assume the responsibility for getting the correct information to the unit clerk in time to meet the 11:30 AM deadline. The three staff nurses who were present agreed with Cathy's point that the burden should be shared by the RNs as well as by the clerks. The two clerks were satisfied. One of them volunteered to report back to the group at the next meeting on how the system is working out.
>
> The next item was another food problem. Viney Carter, a nursing assistant, noted that oftentimes a patient will get his or her food tray just when he or she is about to be taken down for an X-ray. When the patient gets back, the food is cold. Carter stated that it's not a good idea to put the meal back in the warming cart since it's used to store dirty trays before they are taken away. She suggested asking for a small food warmer that would fit into the unit's kitchen and could be used to keep a food tray warm until a transported patient comes back to the unit. Cathy said that

she would suggest the idea to Ivan Edwards, the Clinical Supervisor, and report back to the group next week.

Then Bruce Gould described his experiences at a quality of work life conference that he had been invited to attend as a representative from Parkside. He ran through some of the main themes of the conference. He stated that how to let people design their own work was one of the big issues. 'In one place, a coal mine, everybody learns different jobs. Also they try to make jobs more interesting. In another place, if the work gets finished, workers can go home or stay for education sessions. Here, we might think of what nursing assistants could do to make their jobs more interesting, like getting them involved in patient care conferences or learning more about the technical things.' The nursing assistants nodded in agreement.

Unfortunately, Barnard 5 was an "innovation ghetto" (Toch & Grant, 1982). The weak linkages between the quality of work life project and the sources of institutional authority within the hospital insured that change was encapsulated. There were no real supportive structures for adopting successful outcomes of the Barnard 5 experiment and diffusing them to the rest of the pavilion and to the hospital as a whole.

As we discuss in Chapter 9 it is often difficult for the evaluation researcher to specify the causal factors in the field, where success or failure is difficult to measure and where causal factors are often overdetermined. But in the case described here, the primary cause of the failure to move beyond the boundaries of Barnard 5 was management's refusal to accede legitimacy to a joint project with the unions. The hospital director, Harvey Hertz, did not want to be identified with the project. It was allowed to function, but only within the tacit framework established by Hertz's policy directives. The hospital was entering a period of highly adversarial relations with the largest union in the hospital; the "good old days" of substantial hiring, rapid wage increases, and politically tolerable deficits had come to a close. Given the turbulence of the labor relations climate, it was unrealistic to expect that the QWL project would thrive.

The consultant strategy reflected the lack of management and union ownership of the project and the resultant impotence of the core union-management committee. The consultants saw that the working group on Barnard 5 lacked access to decision makers within the hospital as well as access to important information about the organization, such as the results and implications of the Healthtech staffing survey, that would have allowed the group to work effectively. Given these limits, the consultants decided to make an "end run." They sought out key management figures who were at once sympathetic to the participatory ethos of the project and who enjoyed some measure of autonomy from the hospital director. Dr. Mauer of clinical services seemed a likely figure. He was new, he was recruited to Parkside on the basis of his considerable reputation (and not by Harvey Hertz), and he was well aware of the magnitude of the problems facing him in his role. His relationship to the QWL project was opportunistic, but in a positive sense. He saw the project as a means of gaining visibility, of introducing reforms that, if successful, could build his reputation for innovative management. In turn, the consultants saw him as a contact to a source of real power in the hospital. Moreover, Evans and Meyer saw that many of the problems on Barnard 5 and the other nursing units throughout the hospital were linked to the poor coordination between where patients lived during their hospital stay and departments such as radiology and respiratory therapy where they received clinical treatment. The clinical services project was not only a political plus, it was a response to a critical need.

The proposed training program for Hospital Workers' Union members also addressed a real issue—the reticence and lack of self-confidence of nonprofessional employees. Evans proposed what was essentially a program of assertiveness training for these employees. It is important to keep in mind that the program's main objective—never publicly stated—was to provide a face-saving way of bringing the hospital workers back into the QWL project. It accomplished this objective, but at the cost of using up precious consultant time. From a cost-benefit perspective, it might have been more effective for Edwards and Meyer to have arranged a smaller series of informal sessions with HWU members on the floor. But to do so would have failed to satisfy the political need for the training program.

Given the consultants' intention to stay with the project, their strategy of building widely dispersed "bases" of activity was perhaps one of the few reasonable options open to them. Once they succeeded in building separate constituencies for the project, they could begin the even more difficult process of consolidation. The parts might eventually form a whole. But for now, the structural integrity of the project was lost: There was no central union-management policy-making body, no strategy beyond the opportunistic moves of the consultant team, and no vision of the types of long-term changes that would constitute a successful project.

CHAPTER EIGHT

Maturation and Decline
The Second Half of the Evans Consulation

In the absence of a viable joint union-management steering committee, the Parkside Quality of Work Life Project was not a single entity but a series of loosely connected subprojects—each with different objectives and participants. The structure of the project made sense only from the larger perspective of the consultants' overall strategy—to build ownership for the project among key power figures in the hospital and to improve management capabilities to the point where the fragile gains in communications, intergroup relations, and work procedures that resulted from project activity could be protected. There were essentially five areas of consultant-client activity at Parkside. We will refer to them as subprojects in our assessment in Chapter 10. These include the original pilot project on Barnard 5, the Barnard training program, the "communication network" project (which involved the assistant director of nursing for Barnard Pavilion, the director of nursing, and their respective staffs), the clinical services survey feedback project, and the clinical services/nursing organization mirroring project.

This chapter includes a description of the course of each of these five principal subprojects and covers the period from the late summer of 1977, when it became clear that the steering committee was no longer the focus of consultant activity, to the project's termination a year later. The chapter concludes with an account of the final meeting of the steering committee just prior to termination, impressions of the major participants in the project, and an interpretive summary of the principal events of the second half of the Evans group's tenure in the hospital.

THE BARNARD 5 SUBPROJECT

The conflict between Nancy Marullo and the staff of Barnard 5 over the scheduling of weekend duty was an important turning point in the QWL project. The incident and its aftermath led the consultants to conclude that the small, committed group of RNs on the floor could do little to create lasting reform by themselves. Even with an assistant director of nursing who was more sympathetic to the aims of the project than Nancy Marullo was, it would have been difficult to sustain any major structural innovations on Barnard 5 since so much of the daily rhythm of work activity on the unit was related to other departments and administrative hierarchies. This realization (and the impotence of the steering committee) led the consultants to try to locate supportive managers outside of the hierarchy of nursing.

Thus, apart from the training program for Hospital Workers' Union members, much of the consultants' work on the unit over the second half of the project had the character of a holding action. Two major innovations were in place: the monthly orientation for new residents and weekly staff conferences on the day and evening shifts. Steve Meyer came to the staff conferences occasionally, but scheduling and running them were the responsibility of Cathy Thomas and Ethel Atkins, the senior clinical nurses. There was talk of initiating staff conferences on the night shift but it was never done—perhaps because of the small number of employees who worked nights and because of cross-shift communications problems.

Gradually, the enthusiasm for the project among Barnard 5 staff members began to decline. The participative ethos that had characterized the staff meetings gave way to a business as usual approach in which the senior clinical nurse or clinical supervisor briefed the assembled staff. No longer were the meetings a forum for debating new ideas for changing the nature of work on the unit. In part, the pilot unit project seemed to follow the natural course of so many other participative change projects: without a continual infusion of support from the outside, such projects almost inevitably lose momentum. As Dr. Saltzman described the Barnard 5 project to Steve Meyer: "It's like an engine that's idling; unless things start moving again it's going to die."

But there was also one specific, identifiable reason for the project's decline: the manifest lack of support from outside the unit. As long as staff members limited QWL activity to innovations that required no outside support or approval, such as the dietary form episode described in Chapter 7, there was no problem. But as staff members began to go beyond the "soft" areas of improving communications and fostering more cooperation among different levels of staff on the floor and began to consider reforms that required tangible resources, they were forced to come to terms with their relative powerlessness. One very telling example involved Bruce Gould, the RN who was the most consistently active participant in the Barnard 5 project. Gould came up with the idea of starting a professional library for staff members on the unit. The staff conferences had begun to examine several interesting patient care issues, such as methods of team nursing; and a number of staff members, including nursing assistants, wanted to know more about developments in the field. Gould also had become interested in organizational development—in part because of the project and also through management courses he was taking toward his master's degree in nursing. Gould's proposal—to have a small, open reference library in the staff lounge, where staff members could read during their break periods—received strong support at one of the weekly staff conferences. But the group's request for the library was never honored. No one was sure why the administration failed to respond, although there were some mentions of fears that the books would soon disappear and of the difficulties of buying books and building shelves within the constraints of the existing budget. Later proposals—for the redesign of the nursing station, the renovation of the staff lounge, and the creation of a library of recreational materials for patients—shared a similar fate. After trying (unsuccessfully) to find out why the staff library idea was rejected, Gould and two of the other unit staff members who were active in the QWL project applied for transfers to other areas of the hospital.

By late 1977, the staff conferences were no longer being held on a weekly basis, and it often seemed that it was only the presence of a Columbia research team member that prompted the nurses to call the staff together. Some meetings were little more than briefing sessions— useful, but limited in content and importance. Sometimes the focus of a staff conference was a change in a paperwork requirement. Other sessions were devoted to clinical care questions and were led by nurses from the hospital's in-service training department. There was seldom an explicit reference to the steering committee, the QWL project as a whole, or to abstract issues of labor-management collaboration. No longer were attempts made to promote greater involvement among the nonprofessional staff. When nursing aides and assistants came to meetings, they assumed once again the roles of silent observers, sitting on the periphery, seemingly unconcerned with most of the substantive issues under discussion. The vibrant quality that suffused earlier meetings of the Barnard 5 group had largely disappeared.

THE BARNARD TRAINING PROGRAM

As described earlier, the training program was intended as a means of bringing the hospital workers back into the QWL project. Moe Kurtzman was pleased that Evans and Meyer were making real efforts to build support for the project among nonprofessional personnel, and the training program offered proof that the quality of work life project was a true collaborative effort. But a ten-week training program devoted exclusively to HWU members would be an extremely costly vehicle for making peace with Kurtzman and the union, and it would offer no foreseeable benefits to the other principal constituencies of the project.

With this in mind, the consultants redirected the focus of the program. It now would be open to all staff members on Barnard 5—nurses as well as nonprofessional staff. The initial discussions with Kurtzman were followed by interviews with Nancy Marullo, Ivan Edwards, Sally McBride, and nine members of the Barnard 5 staff. Most of the interviews were conducted by a new member of the consultant team, Dr. John Hampton, a training specialist who was brought in specifically to design and run the program. From his analysis of the interview data, Hampton developed a set of themes that were used to structure the content of the training sessions. Hampton provided an outline of these themes in a memo to the steering committee:

> More effective meetings are needed on Barnard 5. Need to learn to be better meeting planners, leaders and participants.
>
> What to do when there's a problem. Need to learn to raise problems productively so they get resolved rather than resulting in a conflict.
>
> More effective communications: within shifts, across shifts, levels, units and disciplines.
>
> Should develop a climate and attitude of mutual responsibility, respect, cooperation, and teamwork.
>
> Need to increase people's motivation and improve their attitudes.
>
> Must learn to solve disagreements more effectively.
>
> Training should be held away from the unit.
>
> Clarify everyone's job responsibilities.
>
> Death and dying should be included—with the objective of getting the staff to share their feelings about it.

Increased continuity of nursing care.

Human needs are too often disregarded.

How can we find time to be trained when the work load keeps going up.

Hampton and Evans presented the outline and structure of the training program at the thirty-eighth meeting of the steering committee, which took place on October 7, 1977. They ran into problems immediately. Hampton, who held the floor throughout much of the meeting, was unaware of the peculiar dynamics and history of the steering committee. His detailed outline struck a nerve; the program would require a substantial time commitment from the entire nursing unit. The tone of the meeting was sharply reminiscent of the day, months before, when the Wheaton team announced plans for a major off-site training effort—a suggestion that provided the immediate cause for the termination of the contract with Wheaton. After Hampton went through the outline of the training program, Dr. Saltzman started the questioning.

SALTZMAN: "As this group has made it clear before, it is very difficult to get people off the floor. Do we really need ten sessions?"

HAMPTON: (taken aback) "It takes ten sessions to get through the issues brought up in the interviews."

SALTZMAN: "But are these sessions feasible? You want to get all the people off the floor. That's impossible. You need to have constant care on a nursing unit, and it's really even more of a problem when they are so short of staff."

EVANS: (adding a new element to the program) "Right. But we plan to take people from different floors for each session, and we'll offer the sessions more than once."

MARULLO: (to everyone) "Steve talked about having twenty people in the training sessions but at times, there are only twenty-three people working in all of Barnard. There is no way I can take people from other floors to work on Barnard 5. I believe in the *concept* of the training program, but we've got to ask ourselves if it's feasible. There are priorities in his hospital. We can't pay people overtime for this."

HAMPTON: (defensive and angry) "But from my experience you just can't do groups of two or three people."

MARULLO: "Who would be involved in the program?"

HAMPTON: "Nursing staff."

MARULLO: (angrily) "But you've got to make sure that everyone's involved—not just nursing."

The discussion meandered on. Some participants questioned the need for a multisession training program: Was there an alternative? Could the training program be combined with the Barnard 5 staff conferences? Would it make sense to have the hospital's training staff handle the program? In the end, the proposed format of ten two-hour sessions was accepted, but it was clear that, as in so many other activities of the QWL project, there was no defined and interested constituency for the training program. It was no longer a Hospital Workers' Union program, but nursing didn't want it; Evans' attempts to link the program to his work with Marullo failed when she stated that she would not provide the necessary staff release time. (Marullo was under heavy pressure to cut overtime costs.) Even the locus of the program wasn't clear. Was it intended only for Barnard 5 staff, or would it extend to the pavilion as a whole?

The program was finally launched in December of 1977. The results were far different from those envisioned in the original plan. Attendance was a major problem: Only seven of the seventeen invited staff members showed up at the first session, which was devoted to some get-acquainted exercises and team-building activities. After stating that it was impossible to do so, Marullo obtained the needed releases time for the training program. She also provided an enthusiastic introduction to the first session. Unfortunately, in a remark characteristic of her management style, she said angrily: "We're going to find out why so many of the invited people didn't come."

In spite of these shortcomings, participants, including the two Hospital Workers' Union members present (a housekeeping supervisor and a unit clerk from Barnard 5) enjoyed the session. But attendance failed to pick up, and there was little continuity of participation from one week to the next. Staff members came to the program when they could afford the time, although a few were so committed that they came into the sessions on their days off. Hampton, the training consultant, was entertaining. The sessions were fun. But they seemed unrelated to the larger hospital context. Hampton focused on "here and now" problems of Parkside, but the unconnectedness of the training program to the realm of work and authority within the hospital gave it a tone of unreality. In the end, most participants felt that while they had gained personally rewarding knowledge about themselves, it was difficult to see how this knowledge could be applied in the working environment of Parkside.

The Columbia research team's formal evaluation of the training program is presented in Chapter 10.

THE BARNARD "COMMUNICATIONS NETWORK" PROJECT

Evans and Meyer's work with Nancy Marullo intensified after the June 7, 1977 steering committee meeting. No longer was there talk of transferring the center of the project to another pavilion; it was too late to start up again, even if a sympathetic assistant director of nursing could be found elsewhere in the hospital. As described in Chapter 7, the nursing department was in the middle of a major reorganization. At the highest level, reporting relationships between the director of nursing and her leadership group of associate and assistant directors were being changed. The department was also analyzing the relationship between the new first line supervisory positions: senior clinical nurse and clinical supervisor. There was considerable overlap in the responsibilities of these two jobs, and this led to frequent conflicts. The job descriptions were poorly written and failed to solve the tremendous coordination problems that had prompted their creation.

So, as the consultants continued their informal, one-to-one work with Nancy Marullo, it appeared that helping to clarify the roles of the clinical supervisor and senior clinical nurse would be a logical first step in expanding the consultants' presence within the hierarchy of nursing. If they succeeded, the pay-off would be two-fold: first, the consultants would gain a larger measure of legitimacy within the hospital and would raise the status of the quality of work life project as a whole; second, improving supervisor relationships would help reduce the climate of instability that threatened to overwhelm any project-related gains on Barnard 5. It was a creative short-term strategy—one that reflected an understanding of the basic workings of the nursing department.

With Marullo's support, Evans and Meyer held a series of training meetings with the supervisory staff of Barnard Pavilion. They agreed that limiting the scope of this work to Barnard 5 would not be cost effective; the basic problems were pavilionwide. Evans' aim was to develop a "communications network" through weekly meetings of the supervisory personnel within Barnard Pavilion supplemented by meetings with key physicians, including Dr. Saltzman. The specific focus of the group was the troubled relationship between the clinical supervisor and the two or three senior clinical nurses assigned to each of the nursing units.

Steve Meyer assumed the principal consultant role in this project. Much of his time was spent in "role negotiation." He met with the clinical supervisors as a group to clarify their expectations about their roles and how these expectations compared to the actual job description. Then he brought the clinical supervisors and senior clinical nurses together for another round of job clarification. This latter group then met with the assistant director. The iterative process of examining and reassessing different supervisory roles continued till the end of 1977. Marullo was pleased with the results. Once more she had become an enthusiastic client.

But it wasn't clear what effect, if any, this activity had on the status of the QWL project. Marullo continued to insist adamantly that *none* of her work with the consultants was related to the project. In her view, Evans and Meyer were there as management consultants; the fact that their official client was the joint union-management steering committee did not seem to enter her mind. In her view, the project meant time taken away from the pressing issues raised by the reorganization plan, from budgeting, from her attempts to develop a greater sense of her own role. The project also gave employees a forum for griping. Incidents like the scheduling controversy raised expectations without providing the means to satisfy them.

Edwards shared Marullo's perspective. To him, the official project meetings were a burden. The presence of the consultants undercut his authority as a supervisor in that employees went to Evans and Meyer with their problems and concerns rather than him. He lamented that:

> Staff members on the floor feel they are a powerful group because of the project. But you try to do things for these people on the floor and no one is satisfied. It's never enough.

Marullo and Edwards often used the imagery of "we versus they" in describing the QWL project. Their sentiments are echoed by their peers in many other such projects, for it is often the supervisory staff, the "people in the middle," who feel most threatened by participative interventions. Also, Marullo and Edwards were aware that there were no points to be won at Parkside by embracing a project with a union label on it. Thus while Evans and Meyer's work may have reduced the pervasive insecurity about roles within Barnard, it failed to bring the quality of work life project any closer to the centers of power and authority in the hospital.

THE CLINICAL SERVICES SURVEY FEEDBACK PROJECT

The clinical services project got underway in May of 1977 with Dan Hartman's presentation to representatives of twenty departments within the clinical services division. While the meeting was intended for department directors, few actually came. Instead, most sent an administrator or an administrative aide. After the clinical services director's opening remarks, Hartman gave a spirited lecture on the philosophy of survey feedback. His talk was liberally illustrated by success stories drawn from his past consulting experience. Hartman's enthusiasm was infectious, and by the end of the presentation, any initial skepticism had largely dissipated.

As a working session it was less successful, however. The original plan for the meeting called for the distribution of the first round of survey questionnaires and a briefing on the actual mechanics of the survey feedback process. But the questionnaires were not ready yet and it wasn't clear who would be in charge of administration within each department or how or when the questionnaires would be returned for processing. One administrator reacted with dismay when she found out that there was no Spanish version of the questionnaire.

Within two weeks after the meeting, the questionnaires had been distributed to the 1200 employees within the division. Ultimately, 350 of the questionnaires were completed and returned. The response rate varied considerably among the departments and seemed to be related to whether or not a department director showed an interest in the project. Since the survey feedback project was an actual intervention, the Columbia research team was not involved in the administration.

Shortly after the questionnaires were distributed, Dan Hartman left the consultant team over a dispute with Meyer and Evans. Steve Meyer took over the responsibility for the survey feedback project. In July, he and the clinical services director held a series of meetings to organize the timetable for project implementation. Their plan followed a standard feedback model. First, the data would be given to the clinical services director and his senior staff members. Feedback presentations to department heads would follow. Initially, the plan called for one large feedback meeting for all department directors. But later Mauer changed the plan to include a series of meetings with individual department heads. He was concerned that the data would reflect badly on several directors and might create embarrassment or active resistance if displayed in a public forum. The key problem—one that is central to the survey feedback method—was to figure out how to present the data in ways that would not provoke defensiveness, but rather would motivate principals to think about how to use negative findings to improve departmental performance. The next step after the meetings with the department directors would be to set up work teams within each department to identify target problems. This would be followed by general meetings of department employees. Finally, the survey would be readministered in the late fall, and comparisons between the two sets of data would allow for an assessment of the overall project.

It was becoming clear to Meyer and the clinical services director that a project of this magnitude could not be handled by the two of them alone, so plans were made to select and train a small cadre of facilitators—four or five in all—from the administrative ranks of the clinical services division. Facilitators would help work teams to interpret the data, formulate problems to be worked on, and implement corrective changes within a department. To insure that the facilitators were seen as objective and impartial, none would do any facilitation within his or her own department. Each facilitator would be responsible for three or four of the clinical services departments.

Ironically, the facilitator plan increased the time burden for Mauer and Meyer. Recruiting sympathetic and competent facilitators turned out to be a real problem. Mauer's chief administrative aide did not believe in the project and eschewed involvement. Other possible candidates were written off because they lacked the requisite initiative or sensitivity. One notably competent administrator, a young MBA who managed the hospital's renal treatment center, transferred out of the division just after he was selected as a facilitator.

Eventually, the clinical services director assembled a team of four facilitators, and he and Meyer spent a great deal of time training them for the role. But the problems continued. The facilitators discovered that they lacked authority outside of their home departments, and instead of being the "catalysts for change" that their training had led them to believe they would be, they were often regarded as interlopers by physician department directors who wanted no part of the clinical service director's administrative reforms. Some department directors who were sympathetic at first became disillusioned by the slow pace of the project and the substantial time commitment required. A common lament was: "We didn't know what we were getting ourselves in for."

The actual feedback process was chaotic. Some department heads refused to participate, and the data were never used. Others held initial feedback sessions but never got to the next step of forming work teams to begin the actual work of problem solving. Making sense of the data was not easy. Each department was given computer printouts of the raw survey data and crude summary sheets of item scores prepared by Meyer. In most cases, the data were overwhelming and showed few clear patterns. Many were unusable.

Microbiology and the blood bank were singled out as the two departments in which the survey data led to serious attempts at participative reform. But for the rest the data and time constraints posed insurmountable problems. The clinical services director and Meyer held a great many meetings between April and June of 1977 in preparation for department-level feedback meetings in August. But vacation schedules pushed the timetable into the fall, and by then, it was difficult to regain the momentum of the early days of the project. Gradually, the clinical services director began to lose interest. It was clear that the survey feedback project was not going to fulfill his initial hope of improving the management within several of the division's troubled departments, and it was equally clear that he had nothing to gain politically from his continued involvement in the project. Feedback sessions continued sporadically through the spring of 1978, and the second set of questionnaires was administered that May. In the second wave, only 216 questionnaires were returned. The resultant data were never used, nor did the project come to a formal end. It simply disappeared from the agenda of steering committee meetings and as a topic of concern among the consultants. It seemed odd that an enterprise that had involved so many staff and such a substantial commitment of time should fade so quickly and so completely.

THE ORGANIZATION MIRRORING PROJECT

The beginnings of the organization mirroring project go back to the initial discussions between Dan Hartman and the clinical services director in April of 1977. Steve Meyer introduced the concept to staff members on Barnard 5 a month later, but there was little sustained activity over the next few months. Then, gradually, the project gained momentum. Evans and Meyer conducted several interviews with Barnard 5 staff members and employees of the clinical services division to sound out their opinions about an interdepartmental mirroring project. The consultants also produced a mirroring card. The purpose of the card, which was to be distributed to employees on several nursing units and in several of the clinical departments, was to provide a means for employees to express their opinions—positive and negative—about their counterparts in the other division. Blood bank employees, for example, would receive a "mirror image" of themselves as perceived by nursing unit employees. For Evans and Meyer, the mirroring project was a first step in setting up a two-way communications process between the department of nursing and the clinical services division. Their aim was to reduce the antagonism and improve the poor coordination between these two critical functional areas of the hospital. A steering committee made up of clinical services department directors, assistant directors, and other administrative personnel was set up to plan project activities and oversee their implementation. The steering committee included no representatives from either SNA or the HWU.

In late 1977, the steering committee sent out mirroring cards to Barnard 5 and five other nursing units. The card solicited employee opinions about three of the fourteen clinical services departments with substantial contact with nursing floors—the radiology and EKG departments and the blood bank. The initial response rate among nursing unit employees was very low, so the steering committee planned a resurvey. The committee also formulated plans for a pilot project that would involve representatives from a set of nursing units and clinical services departments. Employees would meet in work groups to improve the interface between the two divisions. If the project was successful, it would be expanded to include all nursing units and all of the hospital's clinical services.

Then after the initial planning activity and the mirroring card episode the project languished once more. Evans and Meyer were involved with several other projects during the second half of 1977, including the clinical services survey feedback project and the work with Nancy Marullo, and neither had time for a new venture—especially one that spanned two major divisions of the hospital.

But by the spring of 1978, the consultants were very concerned about what would remain of the QWL project after they left Parkside. From this perspective, the organization mirroring project had a lot to offer. It provided a way to link the consultants' work on the pilot unit, Barnard 5, with their work in nursing and clinical services. It also addressed the need for improvements in coordination along the crucial interface between patient care units and laboratory-based services—a problem area that was now receiving serious attention from senior management. The mirroring project also offered the two consultants an opportunity to use their considerable expertise in improving interpersonal communication.

So in March of 1978, Evans, Meyer, and the heretofore dormant mirroring steering committee worked out a design for pilot projects involving the blood bank and the radiology department. Diversity was the criterion of choice: the blood bank is a small, laboratory-based department with a relatively routine work flow; radiology is a large, complex department with a high volume of activity. But in addition, hospital employees viewed both as problem departments. A typical day on a nursing unit was not complete without at least one missing X-ray photograph or angry phone call to follow up a late blood test or to locate blood that was ordered and never arrived. In short, these two departments had an impact on the quality of work life on nursing units and on patient care as well.

A month later, Evans ran a training session for the employees from blood bank and radiology who had been selected for the pilot project work teams. The session included role-playing problem-solving exercises and techniques for conflict resolution. At meeting's end, the two work teams laid out their meeting schedules and went their separate ways. With the pilot groups now in operation, the mirroring steering committee lacked a salient role. Ostensibly, the group would be the vehicle for diffusing innovations spawned by the work teams, but it would be some time before that stage was reached. The steering committee never met again.

The Radiology Project

The radiology work team held its first task meeting at the end of April of 1978. The team was composed of eight people from radiology and from different nursing units. With Evans' assistance, the team generated a list of problems that were considered important by both radiology and nursing employees. The list included the following:

1. *The Need to Clarify the Meaning of the Term "Stat."* Doctors and nurses used the term loosely and as a means of speeding up the completion of a routine task. Radiology employees felt that the use of "stat" was justified only in emergency situations.

2. *The Lack of a Physician Representative.* The work team concluded that many of the problems discussed involved medical issues and the relationships between doctors, nurses, and the radiology staff. Team members felt the need for a physician representative.

3. *X-ray Procedures.* There were complaints that in some cases, a patient's X-ray procedures were clocked before completion. This resulted in some patients being taken from radiology before all procedures had been carried out properly and fully.

4. *Transporter Time.* The team felt that the waiting time for a transporter to come to pick up a patient and return the patient to a nursing unit was often much too long.

5. *X-ray Delivery.* X-ray reports were delivered to nursing units by messenger. If the patient's medical record was not there, the report would be sent back to radiology. The radiology representatives on the work team felt that someone on the nursing unit should sign for the reports and take responsibility for them until the medical record was sent up to the unit. This would lessen the problem of multiple trips.

6. *Nursing Representation.* The size and membership of the work team fluctuated during its nine-month existence. However, team members complained of radiology overrepresentation and lack of nursing input.

7. *X-ray Requisitions.* Illegible requisitions made it difficult to identify and trace patients.

8. *Improper Filing.* Inpatient X-ray reports were being filed before they were reviewed by the doctor.

9. *Poor Communication and Lack of Knowledge.* Both nursing and radiology representatives felt that they knew very little about the other's division, and that communication was needlessly antagonistic and confused. The team proposed an orientation to the radiology department for nursing staff as a means of dealing with the problem.

10. *Poor Preps.* Radiology representatives complained that the procedures used by nurses to prepare ("prep") a patient for tests were not always done correctly.

11. *Patient Transfers.* When patients were transferred from one nursing unit to another, radiology staff were often confused about where to send reports.

12. *Lost X-ray Photographs.* Physicians sometimes removed X-ray photographs from where they were filed without returning them properly. Effectively, this meant the photograph was lost.

The radiology work team met regularly from April through December of 1978 and alternated between high hopes and much enthusiasm to tremendous frustration over how slowly tasks were moving along. Turnover remained high and the team never succeeded in recruiting a physician member with the commitment of a Dr. Saltzman. On June

20th, the group assessed its progress in the twelve listed problem areas:

KEY: 0 = under discussion
− = not dealt with
+ = action underway

Problem	Action
1. "Stat"	0 Still under discussion.
2. Lack of physician representative	− One was recruited and left. No new prospects.
3. X-ray procedures	+ New procedure installed.
4. Transporter time	0 Plans for a new procedure to be tried in September.
5. X-ray delivery	+ New plan being implemented in all units.
6. Nursing representation	+ Better, though not as much as we would have liked.
7. Illegible X-ray requisitions	− We're going to bring it up to nurses during orientation— it's still a problem.
8. Improper filing	− Still a problem.
9. Radiology-nursing communication	0 In process. A new staff orientation to radiology and orientation for current staff was being planned. Also, copies of the radiology organization chart were being made for nurses.
10. Poor preps	+ Proper procedures for barium enema prep were being written up.
11. Patient transfers	0 To be discussed.
12. Lost X-ray photographs	0 To be discussed.

Based on its assessment, the work team decided that the project was still worth the effort and that it would continue to meet. Slowly, new procedures were suggested and adopted. Radiology staff members arranged a tour for new nursing staff. The work team implemented a new system for dealing with the problem of lost X-ray photographs and improved the procedures for tracking patients. Nurses were given a checklist of the kinds of information required of patients who were sent to radiology.

But as the heavy vacation schedule of the summer months began to cut into attendance, team members became frustrated over unsolved problems, the lack of a physician representative, and what radiology members viewed as a lack of commitment on the part of their colleagues from nursing. In August, the consultants left the hospital.

The team was able to revive some of its earlier spirit in the fall. Instead of trying to solve a dozen problems simultaneously, it focused on one—the delivery of X-ray reports. Team members came up with a new procedure that was designed to eliminate the need for multiple trips to pick up X-ray photos and reports for delivery to the nursing units. The procedure required that residents read the X-rays immediately, sign for them, and turn them over to the unit clerk for insertion into the patient's chart. The project represented a considerable time investment. First, there was a pilot test. Then unit clerks had to be trained in the new procedure, pickup times had to be worked out, the nursing and medical staff had to be briefed, and supervisors had to be persuaded to accept responsibility for helping to correct slip-ups. Those steps involved several months of meetings and discussions. But in the end, the new procedure worked. The work team visited nursing units, examined patients' charts and saw that X-rays now were being read and filed correctly.

Ironically, the work team's success imperiled its existence. Specifically, several team members felt that its goal had been met and it was now time to disband and turn the project over to the steering committee. No one seemed aware that the steering committee had stopped meeting several months before. Other work team members took a process-oriented rather than a task-oriented perspective. They felt that the group had succeeded in opening up lines of communication between two critical divisions of the hospital and that its work should continue. Clearly, this is what Evans and Meyer hoped for before they left the hospital.

In November of 1978, the work team voted to continue its work. A letter was drafted and sent to the chairman of the steering committee. It stated that:

1. The group had met the original goals of the steering committee.
2. "This group process has proved successful as measured by the wide ranging problem solving in both departments . . ."

3. "In having met the original goals, the RNM (radiology-nursing mirroring group) wishes to terminate and reform itself into a permanent committee responsible to the departments of nursing and radiology. The goals of the new committee are:

    a. To expand nursing and medical representation on this committee.

    b. To identify common problems, to seek out and implement solutions, and to monitor the on-going effectiveness of these solutions.

    c. To review proposed program changes from nursing or radiology and to make recommendations regarding the implementation and effect of these changes.

    d. To report to the hospital's senior management group important problems that are beyond the scope of this committee.

    e. To develop communication between nursing and radiology, especially in the areas of staff and in-service education.

    f. To continue to evaluate the effectiveness of this new committee's work.

    Unless the radiology-nursing mirroring subcommittee hears to the contrary, we will reform ourselves by December 14, 1978.

The work team never received a reply to its letter from the steering committee which, as noted, had ceased operations several months before. Despite their expressed intention, the members of the team failed to meet again. The group succumbed to the obvious lack of interest from steering committee representatives and from the senior management of the nursing and clinical services divisions.

The Blood Bank Project

The blood bank work team was formed in April of 1978 at the same time as its radiology counterpart, but its effective life span was considerably shorter—about three months. Members were recruited evenly from blood bank and nursing. The weekly meetings of the team were cochaired by the newly appointed administrator of the blood bank, Phillip Cowell, a former technician, and by William Massing, the assistant director of nursing for the department of psychiatry. Massing was selected because he was available, enthusiastic, and because he was known as an able administrator—qualifications that overrode the limited functional relationship between blood bank and psychiatry.

The eight or so members of the blood bank/nursing work team faced a different set of sociotechnical issues than the radiology team, which saw the sheer size of the radiology department and the difficulties of internal coordinators as paramount concerns. Blood bank's problems were related to its unique mission—the collection, analysis, and storage of human blood. Employees of the blood bank worked within a relatively modern and compact facility that had grown more congested and hectic in recent years due to the escalating need for "blood work." The most critical problems concerned transferring information and units of blood between blood bank and the nursing units. This became the natural focus of the blood bank/nursing organization mirroring work team.

Many of the conflicts between staff members of the two divisions concerned how blood and blood tests were requisitioned. Blood bank staff complained that nurses and unit clerks didn't follow standard procedures; that they often failed to provide the necessary identifying information in their verbal and written requests. Blood would be ordered, prepared, and sent to a nursing unit where it would remain past the expiration period and have to be destroyed—all because no one informed blood bank that a resident had cancelled the order. Blood bank staff also resented the multiple phone calls from different employees on a nursing unit that were related to a single blood order. In turn, the leading complaints from nurses were the discourteous manner of many blood bank employees, errors in the type of blood delivered, and blood arriving late or not at all after being properly requisitioned.

The work team's first step was to set up a method for documenting the sources of routine errors. William Massing, the cochair of the project and director of research for the nursing division, with input from unit clerks, devised a new log sheet for blood bank requisitions. Nursing staff would use the log sheet to order blood; then the log sheet would be sent to the blood bank to be used to document the completion of the order. Both the nursing unit and the blood bank would retain a copy of the sheet. When checking on the status of a blood order, nursing unit personnel could refer to the log sheet to see if the unit clerk—the person who was solely authorized to communicate with the blood bank under the new procedure—had put it in the order in a timely and accurate way. From a behavioral accounting point of view, the proposed new system was ingeniously simple: Improvements in the coordination between blood bank and nursing could be measured by a drop in the number of multiple phone calls and by adherence to the rule that the unit clerk was the sole communications channel to and from nursing units.

The work team came up with several other ideas for improving the coordination between blood bank and the nursing units. Representatives from blood bank were invited to speak at nursing staff meetings and the orientation for newly hired nursing graduates. In return, William Massing briefed blood bank staff on the nursing department reorganization. Other suggestions included printing a blood bank news bulletin that would be distributed on a regular basis to nursing floors. Bill Evans, who served as a process consultant in several of these meetings, convinced the group to hold off on these and other longer-term projects until the new log form and related procedures had been given a thorough tryout.

The work team decided to test the log form on the nursing floors within psychiatry—a department with limited blood demands. The team's strategy was to start small and expand gradually to areas of greater demand within the hospital. Unit clerks in psychiatry were given an orientation to the new log procedures; a one-month trial period followed.

After the month was over, the work team met with the unit clerks and Phillip Cowell, the administrative director of the blood bank, to evaluate the results. All were enthusiastic about the trial project, including the unit clerks who would bear much of the additional responsibility engendered by the new procedures. (Shortly after the meeting, the procedure was modified, and RNs were included as authorized callers since a unit clerk was not always on duty.) The work team prepared a humorous skit that would be delivered as part of a blood bank "road show" to all nursing units that participated in the project. The project cochair, William Massing, and several staff members from nursing floors were invited to the blood bank for the opening performance. The script went as follows:

Set:	Two desks, two telephones, two spotlights.
Scene opens:	Spotlight on staff nurse who is seated at desk checking patient's charts. She snaps her fingers, picks up the phone and calls blood bank.
	Second light illuminates desk where blood bank registrar is busy tagging bloods.
	Ring, ring, ring, ring. Registrar is busy with the blood. Nurse initiating the call begins to show impatience. Tapping fingers on desk.
REGISTRAR:	(Still not finished tagging) Blood Bank, hold please. (She places the phone on hold and completes the tagging of blood.)

NURSE:	Hello, this is . . . (Shows obvious annoyance at being placed on hold.) Damn! (Drums her fingers on desk.)
REGISTRAR:	Sorry to keep you waiting, may I help you?
NURSE:	This is Miss Pollack from the ICU. Can you tell me if you have a group and Rh on a patient of ours, James Sterling?
REGISTRAR:	Can you give me Mr. Sterling's unit number?
NURSE:	Sure, just a moment. (She rummages through several articles on the desk. Meanwhile the registrar is showing her impatience.)
REGISTRAR:	(Speaking to herself.) Why can't they have the unit number when they call?
NURSE:	Mr. Sterling's unit number is 1234567.
REGISTRAR:	(Looking through a log on her desk.) Yes, we have a group and Rh on James Sterling.
NURSE:	Thank you. (Hangs up, making notation on chart.) (registrar hangs up.)

Both spotlights fade out.

| NARRATOR: | What we've just witnessed was the needless sowing of the seeds of animosity between a nursing care unit and the blood bank. Two hours have passed since the initial inquiry. It is now 11:00 AM. |

(Spotlight on the nurse; she picks up the phone and dials blood bank. Ring, ring, ring.)

REGISTRAR:	Blood Bank, Mrs. Geist.
NURSE:	Can I send a messenger to pick up a unit of blood for Mr. James Sterling?
REGISTRAR:	One moment please. (She checks log on desk twice.) We don't have blood reserved for James Sterling.
NURSE:	(Showing slight irritation) Would you check again? I'm sure we have blood for Sterling. (Exasperated.)
REGISTRAR:	(Annoyed) I've already looked twice. We don't have blood for Sterling. (Firmly.)
NURSE:	This is ridiculous, I myself personally called the blood bank around 9:00 AM. I asked if you had a group and Rh

on James Sterling. (Incredulously.) Some one there told me you did!

REGISTRAR: That's right, I recall the conversation. I was the person you spoke to earlier. We do have a group and Rh on Sterling. Sterling is group A Rh Positive.

NURSE: When I asked if you had a group and Rh, I assumed you knew I was referring to blood held on reserve for this patient.

REGISTRAR: We handle hundreds of specimens a day. Some are for group and Rh only, some are for compatibility tests and reservation. You asked a question, I gave you an answer. If you want blood placed on reserve you'll have to send requisition slips.

NURSE: How many slips for three units of packed cells? And how long will it take? I told the doctor blood was ready in the blood bank.

REGISTRAR: Send down one requisition for each unit of whole blood or packed cells. It will take between one to two hours before the blood is available.

NURSE: (Reaching for requisitions while hanging up the phone) Damn!

NARRATOR: What we've just witnessed, to borrow a phrase from a recent movie, is an example of "a failure to communicate." The Nurse used a phrase "group and Rh." Her interpretation of the phrase "group and Rh," as we noticed, did not exactly coincide with that of the blood bank registrar. The battle lines are drawn. But most importantly our patient, Mr. Sterling, will experience an unnecessary two-hour delay before he receives his blood transfusion. With just a slight modification of the previous scene we might very easily have saved a few hard feelings, and we most definitively would have eliminated a two-hour delay in rendering patient care. Let's take another look at our little scene.

Repeat initial opening. (This time nurse has addressograph card.)
Ring, ring, ring, ring as in opening scene.

REGISTRAR: (Still not finished tagging) Good morning, Blood Bank, Mrs. Geist.

NURSE: Good morning, this is Miss Pollack from the ICU. Do you have blood reserved for Mr. James Sterling?

REGISTRAR: Would you hold for a moment please? (Places call on hold, finishes tagging blood) Sorry for the delay, what was the patient's name and unit number?

NURSE: The patient is James Sterling, unit number, 1234567. (with addressograph card)

REGISTRAR: (After checking log) Hello, we have a group and Rh only on Mr. Sterling. If you would like compatibility tests done and blood placed on reserve, send down requisitions.

NURSE: I'm sending three requisitions for packed cells. How long will it take until the blood is available?

REGISTRAR: The blood should be ready between one to two hours.

NURSE: We'll call to confirm and send a messenger to pick up the blood at around 11:00 AM.

Lights fade out.

NARRATOR: The bottom line: The patient received his prescribed therapy two hours sooner.

              The variable which facilitated better patient care was merely the extension of simple telephone courtesy by the blood bank's registrar, coupled with the utilization, by the nurse, of concise and precise terminology.

On July 25, the mirroring work team met to review the data that had been collected in the pilot trial. In the intervening month, the project had been expanded to four nursing units including one that was outside the department of psychiatry. The work team also chose eight nursing units as "controls." The criteria for selecting them and their characteristics were never made clear. The data, presented in the form of a tally sheet, seemed to participants to indicate that the project was an unqualified success. Specifically, only three of the ninety-five calls that were monitored over a two-week period were categorized as repeat calls, that is, calls made for the purpose of tracking an errant blood order. Some of the staff members present expressed concerns about the home-grown evaluation procedures used in the study. And most had difficulty in interpreting the data apart from the bottom line figure of only three repeat calls. Nonetheless, the project demonstrated that staff members from two antagonistic divisions of the hospital could come together and make concrete improvements in work procedures—

improvements that eased the routine tension on both ends of the telephone and resulted in better patient care. In its own way, the blood
bank project was the kind of activity that the Parkside Quality of
Work Life Project was intended to promote.

Thus it is all the more surprising (and depressing) that the mirroring working group never met again after July 25. The project never
terminated formally; log forms continued to drift in sporadically from
the nursing units. They were kept dutifully but never used. By the following November, the project had, in effect, disappeared. The senior
supervisor of the blood bank, who was interviewed at that time by a
Columbia research team member, reported that while the project did
reduce the frequency of multiple telephone calls to the blood bank for a
while, the problem had returned.

The blood bank project illustrates one of the major concerns of quality of work life advocates—that QWL interventions, even successful
ones, are often fragile and short-lived. The work team developed to the
point where it could propose, implement and (however crudely) measure the results of its own interventions. Throughout the three-month
operating period of the group, Bill Evans remained in the background.
His manifest role was limited to helping the group to clarify its goals,
to consider the implications of different courses of action, and to keep
moving. But Evans also provided legitimacy. His presence conveyed
the message that participative planning and decision making—highly
unusual in the context of Parkside—were acceptable despite the lack
of support from senior management. When Evans' contract ended the
week after the July 25 meeting, so did the sanction needed to keep the
project alive.

THE PARKSIDE QUALITY OF WORK LIFE PROJECT COMES TO AN END

On July 6, 1978, Evans and Meyer scheduled a final meeting of the
Parkside Quality of Work Life Project Steering Committee to review
the accomplishments of the project and to present plans for diffusing
project activities after the official termination date, August 31. Although the meeting was called for 1:30, members of the steering
committee did not begin to arrive until almost 2:00. Blanche Reiner,
Nancy Marullo, and Ivan Edwards arrived first and were followed
about ten minutes later by another group which included Jack Mauer,
Meredith Klein, a representative from personnel and training (who
had replaced Loretta Musial on the committee), and Cathy Thomas
from Barnard 5.

In their summary briefing, Evans and Meyer stressed the positive aspects of the project. Evans recounted the major project activities: The Barnard 5 staff conferences had continued successfully and would be expanded to include the night shift; the monthly orientation sessions for new residents on the unit had continued; the organization mirroring project had had mixed results—the blood bank project had been successful, but the radiology department project had stalled—because of difficulties in getting physician involvement. The communications network project within the nursing department hierarchy in Barnard Pavilion had made progress in clarifying supervisory roles and relationships. After Evans finished, Cathy Thomas, the day senior clinical nurse from Barnard 5, added some comments that supported Evans' positive assessment. She noted that the staff conferences were held every week and that many levels of staff were participating, although Hospital Workers' Union members still remained less vocal than others. The blood bank project had made a "real difference," she said. Then Ivan Edwards commented that he was using the staff meetings to orient the seven new RNs who had been assigned to Barnard 5.

Meredith Klein, who spoke next, continued the positive tone of the meeting. She remarked that the staff conferences and residents' orientation would become standard practice throughout the hospital, though she said little about how diffusion of these innovations would be handled administratively. The results of the organization mirroring project would be presented to the hospital's senior management group; she hoped that the group would adopt the concept on a hospitalwide basis. She noted that several nurses and nursing administrators had expressed interest in hearing more about the Barnard 5 project— implying that it had become institutionalized to the point that other areas of the hospital were thinking about starting their own QWL activities. She concluded by noting that Evans' work with her leadership group had been very helpful in clarifying the process of change within the department of nursing.

Up to this point, no one had commented on the fact that there was not a single union representative at the meeting, nor did Moe Kurtzman or Sally McBride leave word about why they would not be able to attend. Finally, Blanche Reiner offered a comment that she had made in one form or another throughout the project: "All this is good but we've got to involve the hospital workers in this." Evans responded in a tone that reflected his considerable frustration over this issue:

> I don't think you ever got the support from the hospital workers that you needed. Moe has been cooperative, but he was not an active participant.

The responsibility for many of these potential changes must fall to management. Some things have been good, and the hospital is picking up on them. But collaboration with the union presents problems. It would be a mistake not to involve the union, but not at this level. It's better to get involvement at the unit level.

Evans ended the hour-and-a-half-long meeting by briefly reviewing the specific recommendations of the consultants for the diffusion of project activities. The recommendations are listed in Table 8.1.

Officially, the project continued through the end of the month, but the steering committee meeting marked the last on-site visit by the consultants and the effective end of the project.

EPILOGUE

The authors returned to Parkside seven months later, in February of 1979, to find out if the committments made at the July termination meeting had been kept. We found that the steering committee never reconvened, and that Evans' recommendations were never implemented. Only the activities on Barnard 5, specifically the residents' orientation and the staff conferences, continued, although sporadically.

We found that many of the principal figures involved in the QWL project had left the hospital or were planning to leave soon. Dr. Saltzman was about to become the director of a smaller suburban hospital. He summed up his assessment of the project in a long interview:

> To tell you the truth I don't even know if they are still having their weekly staff meetings on Barnard 5. I still meet with Marullo and all her supervisory staff—we meet once a month and talk about problems that involve patient care, admissions, and discharges. I never felt that the quality of work program changed that one bit.

> My gut feeling is that the project did something while it was going on but what it left behind was minimal. Unless the senior management of the hospital change their attitudes about the personnel here, things aren't going to change. This sort of thing was like a little tempest in a teapot, boiling away. But as soon as they turned off the flame, the bubbling stopped.

Moe Kurtzman offered a similar assessment:

> Lasting effects? I don't know. It's mired, and it's going to die. The only lasting effect is the money that's been spent on the project. It will have a lasting effect on Bill Evans and Associates' pockets.

Table 8.1. Consultants' Recommendations to Quality of Work Life Project Steering Committee

Specific Recommendations

Subject	Diffusion Activity		Person Responsible	
Staff Conferences	A.	Train senior clinical nurses or supervisor to conduct staff conferences.	A.	Assistant director of nursing for research and training.
	B.	Spread staff conferences by pavilion.	B.	Assistant director of nursing should provide support and leadership.
	C.	Assistant director of nursing meet bimonthly with supervisors to check how staff conferences progressing and share ideas that have emerged in conferences.	C.	Assistant director of nursing call and conduct bimonthly meetings.
	D.	Monthly, shifts conduct joint staff conferences.	D.	Senior clinical nurses or clinical supervisors.
Doctor's Orientation	A.	Conduct orientation in surgical division (Saltzman, Marullo proposal).	A.	Dr. Saltzman and Barnard Assistant Director of Nursing.
	B.	Based on surgical experience recommend for hospital wide use where appropriate	B.	Dr. Saltzman and Director of Nursing Klein.
Organization Mirroring	A.	Evaluate results of test.	A.	Director of nursing and clinical services director.
	B.	Based on results, expand number of areas conducting organization mirroring activities.	B.	Director of nursing and clinical services director.
		1. Present results and needed training to nursing and clinical services people		1. Use past participants in organization mirroring.

	2. Identify steering committee or coproject directors to help diffuse activity and solve hospital wide issues.	2. Appointees of the directors of nursing and clinical services.
	3. Steering committee or coproject director develop protocol for solving problems in organization mirroring groups.	3. Project steering committee.
Leadership Training A. Running staff conferences.		4. Assistant directors of nursing should provide leadership. Assistant director of nursing for research and training should provide training.
B. Basic problem-solving methods		
C. Decision making (when to involve others).		
D. Interpersonal conflict resolution.		
E. Problem identification self diagnosis (force field analysis).		
F. Communications—Listing/feedback		
Responsibilities Clarification A. Continue to clarify responsibilities of unit leadership down to and including staff on unit.		Director of nursing and the assistant directors of nursing.
Communications Network A. Implement a communications network on all floors. (Dr. Saltzman/Marullo model).		Physician and assistant director of nursing.
Attitude Survey and Feedback Process A. If the survey continues to be viewed as useful, it should be done periodically and perhaps expanded to other parts of the hospital.		Director of clinical services.

Nancy Marullo and Jack Mauer, the other two members of the steering committee working group, left the hospital after the termination of the project and were not interviewed.

It is fitting to end this history of the Parkside Quality of Work Life Project with the words of Bruce Gould, who over the three-year history of the project, remained its most committed participant.

> Sure, I felt I changed because of the project. Before, I felt reluctant to say things to the doctors, to tell them that there were certain things that I expected of them just as they expected things of me as a nurse. Now, I say what's on my mind. I look around and I can see this in other people, too. There is more pride in the floor now—a sense that this is our floor, that there is something special about Barnard 5. I'm not sure the nursing aides would agree with this, I haven't talked to them. But it's certainly true for the nurses.
>
> But I'm afraid that it's in danger of being lost. So far, we've hung on to it, but a lot of it has to do with me and with Cathy Thomas. And now she's transferred to the night shift. The doctors are a little more conscientious about not leaving stuff around, and they have a little more respect for the people on the floor. But people don't take it upon themselves to do the work required to keep this project going. If I say: 'OK, we're having an orientation,' people will come. But if I wasn't here, I don't know who would carry it on.

INTERPRETIVE SUMMARY

By the tenth month of the project, in June of 1977, the Evans consultant team had concluded that the joint labor-management steering committee would never be an effective policy-making group. Several committee members held only marginally important positions in the hospital and could provide little support for QWL activity on Barnard 5. The more powerful members of the committee, including director of nursing Meredith Klein, chose not to exercise their authority in the service of the QWL project. So, while the steering committee remained the official client of the consultant team, the real focus of attention of Evans and his colleagues turned elsewhere in the hospital. In this chapter, we described the consultants' efforts to develop ties between the QWL project and strategically important managers. In this concluding summary, we will outline the three major objectives of the consultants' strategy and the obstacles that ultimately led to their failure to meet these objectives. We conclude with a brief discussion of problems that emerged during the course of the Parkside Project that have surfaced in other QWL projects as well.

Evans and his colleagues evolved a strategy around three objectives, described here in order of increasing specificity:

1. *Increase the legitimacy of the Quality of Work Life Project at Parkside.* The consultants saw that the project was not centrally important to management and the unions. It had symbolic value to both sides—as a public affirmation of the patient care mission and concern for employee well-being—but neither management nor the unions felt sufficient ownership over the project to commit the resources necessary to make it work in ways that would begin to justify the considerable monetary costs involved. Evans and Meyer's response was to seek out and "convert" individual managers to the QWL cause while quietly drawing in the leadership of the Hospital Workers' Union.

2. *Provide training to the nursing administration hierarchy of Barnard Pavilion.* The consultants decided that it was not feasible to transfer the project to another nursing care pavilion in spite of the fact that the assistant director for nursing in Barnard, Nancy Marullo, was an extremely difficult client to work with. There was simply not enough time to build a base of support outside of Barnard. Given this fact, they decided to improve the management performance of the nursing administration of Barnard Pavilion. The consultants reasoned that this would improve the likelihood that innovations on Barnard 5 would survive and be adopted on other nursing units.

3. *Improve the capabilities of the assistant director of nursing in Barnard Pavilion.* Nancy Marullo was very insecure as a manager. As a member of the Columbia research team expressed the problem in an internal memo to the research staff: "Marullo sees power slipping through her hands. She wants to grasp it and keep it from getting away. She's not the type for participative management." The consultants' strategy was to help her increase her basic competence as a manager and by so doing, increase her capacity for accepting a more democratic managerial style.

Overall, the consultants' strategy was to locate sympathetic managers in positions of authority who could be counted on to make a commitment to the project, to win the support of the principal union, to build a supportive environment for QWL within Barnard Pavilion, to train individual managers, and to weave the QWL project into the ongoing activities of the hospital. As strategists, the consultants deserve high marks for their efforts. They diagnosed correctly a difficult situation and came up with a rational plan for increasing the viability of the project. But in the end, they failed to win the support necessary to sustain the QWL project beyond its official termination date. When the project budget was exhausted, the consultants left the hospital, and their diffusion plans went with them.

The course of the Barnard communications network subproject is illustrative of what the consultants were up against. The subproject was successful in building credibility for the consultant team and also responded to a real need—to provide clarification of the roles of nursing administrators within Barnard Pavilion. In the case of Evans' work with the director of nursing, role clarification extended to the highest administrative level within the nursing department. While Marullo and Klein felt that Evans and Meyer were helpful, the consultants' work did not lead to a closer relationship between the two administrators and the QWL project. Marullo in particular made a clear distinction between Evans and Meyer's training sessions with her administrative hierarchy and their attempts to involve her in the QWL project. The project was kept isolated from the central arena of organizational change for one important reason: The director of the hospital had given clear signs that union-management cooperation was incompatible with management's short-term strategy for putting the hospital on a better fiscal footing. The policy was never articulated openly, but in the intensely political environment of the hospital, the message to subordinates was abundantly clear.

The size and complexity of the hospital were also factors in the course of the implementation of the consultants' strategy. On the one hand, Evans and Meyer had the freedom to roam about and search for sympathetic clients while maintaining Barnard 5 as a base of operations. But this led the consultants further away from the original concept of a joint union-management endeavor that would involve lower level employees in basic decisions about the work life of units and departments. The size of the hospital also caused the consultants to stretch their resources to the point where their effectiveness in any one of the five major subprojects was seriously compromised. The most serious problems were posed by the clinical services survey feedback project, which included initially twenty departments and over 1200 employees. The project finally proved to be unworkable. By the end of the QWL project, the consultants appeared to have no overriding conception of what a successful project would involve. Their energy had been spent in trying to build supportive constituencies for the project, but eventually time ran out. And the steering committee never had a coherent picture of how Parkside would be different if the project worked. Lawler's (1982) point about the value of an organizing metaphor of change is most relevant here. He notes that:

In . . . successful projects, key participants typically share a vision of the desired end state. In . . . unsuccessful projects, the participants rarely have a clear idea of where they would like to take the organization, and they tend to lack a clear overview of how all the pieces fit together. In short, they tend to see the forests, not the trees. [p. 310]

The Parkside Quality of Work Life Project also encountered problems that have been commonly reported by many who have participated in or carried out research on QWL projects. Considerable recent attention has focused on the question of institutionalization of the outcomes of QWL projects. The evidence that is available is rather depressing. Even projects that are deemed successful by participants seldom survive for five or more years.

At Parkside, QWL reform was sanctioned by an agreement that pledged management and the unions to support employee initiatives for improving the quality of work life and patient care. Change was facilitated by a team of consultants with excellent reputations in areas of interpersonal relations, training, and organization diagnosis. For a period of time, in some areas of project activity—namely the original experimental unit, Barnard 5, and in the blood bank and department of radiology—employee involvement led to significant improvements in the organization of work and the quality of work life. What characterized all three of these sites was that employees were given an opportunity to identify concrete problems affecting their daily work lives and to solve these problems by using their own collectively derived ideas. A critical factor here is the sense of ownership that emerged as employees began to experiment with new ideas; in all three of the cases, employees spoke of "our" project.

But despite the manifest enthusiasm for the collaborative process of QWL, none of the projects was institutionalized. The lesson here is that even successful employee involvement efforts have little chance of surviving without visible, direct support from those in positions of authority. Allowing QWL to happen is not enough; in a short time, employees within a specific work unit exhaust possibilities for bringing about change within the boundaries of the unit. Attention turns inevitably to the unit's relationship to higher levels in the organization and to problems that, to be solved, must involve upper management. At Parkside, higher level support was not there. When this became clear to employees, site-level QWL structures—such as the joint mirroring committees—quickly collapsed.

Another common problem of QWL programs is the difficulty in winning the support of middle management and first-line supervisors. At Parkside, this problem is clearly shown in the attitudes and behavior of the assistant director of nursing for Barnard Pavilion, Nancy Marullo, and the clinical supervisor for Barnard 5, Ivan Edwards. Both saw the project as a burden. They felt that QWL-related activities wasted precious time and created staff expectations for changes that were totally unrealistic. They believed that the presence of the consultants undercut their own relationships with staff members. The consultants were sensitive to these complaints, but in the end it is doubtful whether they were able to make Marullo and Edwards any more sympathetic to the project. In retrospect, it is not difficult to see why the two Parkside figures took a critical position. They were assigned considerable responsibility for the implementation of the project within Barnard—everything from arranging release time for employees to holding meetings to air employee grievances—and the project was not for them but rather for the employees and, as much as it functioned, for the joint union-management steering committee. What Marullo and Edwards would gain from the project was never made clear.

CHAPTER NINE

Assessment Methods

The methods section of an empirical field research effort typically describes the different instruments, data collection strategies, and sample characteristics relevant to the study. It usually presents a carefully planned and rational approach to measurement that was implemented with few if any problems. The section is, therefore, normally a factual, technical, and uneventful description of the implementation of a predetermined measurement and analysis strategy.

However, we have found that such terse descriptions of research methods are frequently post hoc reconstructions of how the research was conducted. They are an attempt to make sense of a series of events that occurred within an uncertain and ambiguous environment. They reflect the fact that researchers, as human beings, strive to make sense of their behavior and to develop explanations of their activities, sometimes after the fact. Many times, field research in organizations is much more organic, unplanned, and even anarchic than written reports indicate. Indeed, it can be argued that the effectiveness of some research may lie in its evolutionary nature, much as the effectiveness of an organization may be a function of its disorganization and ambiguity (Weick, 1977).

Whether or not field research is more effective when preplanned is irrelevant here. The important point is that the nature of the research effort be accurately communicated so that others can evaluate the research results, understand how the research was actually carried out, and, if desired, duplicate the work.

This chapter will seek to accurately communicate our general assessment strategy. It will attempt to communicate how the assessment actually evolved over time. The focus will be on the general question of how to assess the project as a whole over the period of three years,

155

rather than on details such as the psychometric properties of question-naire scales or similar material. Those matters will be dealt with in Chapter 10.

ORGANIZATIONAL RESEARCH IN THE FIELD

Field research in organizations poses a series of challenges and problems to the researcher attempting to use traditional scientific methods. The researcher enters into an ongoing stream of behavior to generate and collect data related to the development of knowledge. The entry of a researcher into the life of an organization, however, is not a neutral event. Measurement constitutes a potentially significant activity in organizational life and thus may spur a variety of reactions by the organization's members (Argyris, 1952; Schatzman & Strauss, 1973; Lawler, Nadler &, Cammann, 1980; Seashore & Mirvis, 1983). While these reactions are, in themselves, additional data about the nature of organizational life, they do pose problems in the collection of valid and reliable information.

The field experiment involving the active manipulation of organizational variables poses even more complex issues (Seashore, 1964; Barnes, 1967). An experiment is a research strategy for determining the link between constructs by the manipulation of certain variables and the observation of a larger set of variables within a controlled situation. The manipulation is another potentially significant disruption of the normal stream of behavior and thus may result in many unpredicted outcomes. The issue of subject reactions is thus heightened. In addition, there is a tremendous problem regarding control. Since organizations are dynamic, changes occur over time (both internal and external to the organization) which affect the conditions of the experiment, confound the data, and interfere with the experimental manipulation, thereby distorting the research's original thrust. Many would argue that these "interferences" are in reality the phenomena that are interesting, and that they should be viewed as opportunities for generating additional data (and the authors agree with this position). However, the fact remains that the unplanned and unpredicted events that affect the experimental design in the field make it much more difficult to fashion unambiguous interpretations of the data collected.

The Parkside Quality of Work Life Project was plagued (or blessed, depending upon one's perspective) with these typical problems of field research and experimentation. In addition, three other conditions of the project made the measurement and assessment task more complex.

First, the project occurred over a long period of time. The initial formal meetings of all of the parties occurred in May of 1975, and the final on-site measurement activities of the research team took place in December of 1978. Interviews with key participants were conducted in February of 1979. The researchers and project participants were thus actively involved in the project for over three and a half years. This extended involvement, while yielding rich data about an organization over time, added to the problems of data collection and inference because of factors such as researcher fatigue, the increased range of possible intervening variables (ranging from strikes to personnel changes to macroeconomic factors) and so on.

Second, the consultation developed in an evolutionary rather than preplanned fashion. The consultants* did not lay out a plan for changes and then implement that plan. Rather, they were involved in incremental decision making; they formed key strategic decisions as opportunities or demands were presented to them. Therefore the researchers found it difficult to anticipate the consultant activities and prepare in advance criteria for measurement.

Third, the project did not have demonstrable success. This influenced the feelings of the people in the organization (and the researchers) towards the project and thus affected the nature and scope of data collected.

All three of these factors were critical determinants of the nature of the research and assessment activities at Parkside. In the remainder of this chapter, we will constantly refer to these fundamental influences on the conduct of the research.

Within this context, we will describe the research effort in two major sections. In the first, we will outline the general assessment strategy. In particular, the original strategy will be described and then contrasted with the strategy which later evolved. In the second, we will identify and discuss some critical problems encountered by the assessment team in implementing its evolutionary strategy. As mentioned earlier, the specific characteristics of the measurement instruments and data analysis procedures will be described later, in the particular sections on each of the distinct subprojects in Chapter 10.

---

*As the narrative chapters describe, there were two consultant teams involved in the Parkside project. The first team, Wheaton Associates, was dismissed after several months. Much of the assessment strategy was developed during the two-year tenure of the Evans consulting group.

THE EVOLUTION OF A GENERAL ASSESSMENT STRATEGY

Assumptions of the Original Project Strategy

The assessment component of the project was originally based on a standardized approach to assessment of organizational change developed for the various projects that made up the Michigan Quality of Work Program. At its core was the Michigan Organization Assessment Package (Lawler, Nadler, & Mirvis, 1983), a set of instruments and procedures developed at the University of Michigan's Institute for Social Research for the assessment of organizational changes such as those contemplated in the various QWL projects.

The Michigan package was based on five assumptions about the conduct of research at the different QWL sites. These assumptions were as follows:

1. *Known and Bounded Experimental Unit.* It was assumed that the experimental unit in each project would be identified ahead of time, and that it would be relatively stable for most of the project's duration. It was also assumed that the experimental unit could be clearly identified, that the boundaries between it and other units would be distinct. Thus once the unit was identified, measurement could take place before the consultation work started and would provide stable baseline data about the experimental unit before any intervention.

2. *Known and Clear Consulting Strategy.* It was assumed that early in the project the consultants would be able to identify their consulting strategy and planned activities and would be able to predict the outcomes of their work. While this would not be possible immediately, it was assumed that the consultants would be able to make such plans and predictions after doing their initial diagnostic work. The clear and identified consulting strategy would allow researchers a clear focus for their evaluation of consultant activities and outcomes. In addition, the consultant's predictions of outcomes would serve as hypotheses to be tested by the researchers. This would help the latter to distinguish between planned changes in outcomes and either chance variation or variation resulting from events unrelated to the consultation.

3. *Accurate and Available Performance Measures.* The researchers wanted to measure a variety of project outcomes, not just employees' reports on their own attitudes and perceptions. For this reason, the Michigan package called for data collection about various

"performance"measures, including data on and indicators of employee behavior and productivity of the work units in question. The assumption was that accurate and reliable measures of the performance being examined would be feasible, and that such data would be collected by the organization as part of standard information and control systems. As a result, these data would be in a retrievable form.

4. *Comparable and Uncontaminated Control Groups.* Each unit-level project was planned to be an experiment, rather than merely a case study. Therefore it was assumed that for each experimental unit at the focus of consulting activity, a comparable control (or comparison) unit not involved in project activity would also be measured. The assumption was that comparable units could be identified through either random selection or matching, that these control units would not be affected by the project activities in the experimental unit and that the number of subjects and subunits in the experimental and control units would be adequate for statistical analyses of differences over time.

5. *Supportive QWL Structure.* It was anticipated that data collection in the field in the context of a joint labor-management project might be difficult. However, it was assumed that the QWL project structure (including the various QWL committees) would support the research activity, much as the structure would support the consultation. The QWL committees, it was expected, would be interested in collecting and analyzing data about the project so that they could decide what innovations to discontinue or modify. The generation, collection, analysis, and reporting of valid data was perceived to be in everyone's interest. It was also mandated by the funding arrangement.

Based on these assumptions, a general measurement strategy was developed. In particular, the Michigan package described what was called a broad *measurement net* to be implemented in the experimental and control units prior to any consultant activity. That net would be wide enough to pick up most effects of any of the types of interventions envisioned. It was anticipated that this general net would be augmented with additional data collection devices as soon as the consulting strategy (and thus the experimental hypotheses) became evident.

The package consisted of three major types of instrumentation. First, a questionnaire was developed to determine employee attitudes and perceptions. The Michigan Organizational Assessment Questionnaire (Cammann, Fichman, Jenkins & Klesh, 1983) included a number of different component modules focusing on specific sets of variables, such as individual differences, individual expectancies, perceptions of job characteristics, perceptions of supervisory behavior, levels of influence in decision making, and perceptions of labor-management relations.

Second, the package included guidelines for the identification and collection of employee and organizational performance data. These "behavioral-economic" measures (Macy & Mirvis, 1983) were designed to obtain objective measures of the consultation's effects.

Finally, the package included a guide for observation of the projects. It laid out some general principles for observation, suggested some approaches, and established some role relationships but did not include any specific instrumentation. In total, the package provided a set of multimethod data collection technologies for measurement and assessment of the projects.

Actual Conditions at Parkside

As planned, the measurement package was implemented in a variety of QWL sites. However, at Parkside problems occurred from the start. They concerned the nature, scope, and operation of the measurement activity. In particular, many of the actual site conditions differed significantly from those assumed in the package design. (See Table 9.1 for a comparison of the assumed and actual conditions for research.) The actual conditions at the site were as follows:

1. *Changing Focal Units with Unclear Boundaries.* During the project, the focal point of QWL activity changed. Originally, the focal unit was the pilot surgical unit, and most of the measures were con-

Table 9.1.   Assumed Versus Actual Conditions for Research at Parkside

Conditions assumed for original research strategy	Actual conditions at the site
1. A known and bounded experimental unit	1. Constant changes in the focal unit; unclear and ambiguous boundaries among units
2. A known and clear consulting strategy	2. Shifting, ambiguous, consulting strategy
3. Available and accurate performance measures.	3. Inaccessible or nonexistent performance measures.
4. Comparable and uncontaminated control groups	4. Noncomparable and contaminated control groups
5. A QWL structure to support the assessment work	5. A weak QWL structure which provided little support

structed to ascertain changes in that unit. However, several months after the second consulting team began its work, emphasis shifted to the hospital's clinical services departments. At the same time, work began at the supervisory level of the pilot unit (nursing supervision at the pavilion level and physicians). This meant dealing with the team reporting to the director of nursing. Similarly, the organizational mirroring subproject included a set of patient care units linked to two departments in clinical services. Thus the original focus on the pilot surgical unit widened to involve the pavilion, the nursing department, the clinical services departments, and selected physicians and administrators.

In addition, the boundaries of the units were somewhat unclear. In particular, the staffing patterns made it difficult to determine the membership of a particular focal unit. For example, on the pilot unit, besides the core nursing staff, there were also attending physicians who had patients on other hospital units and affiliations on other floors. Technicians frequently appeared on the floor to provide specific services, but they also worked on other floors. Residents were assigned to the floor for only three months at a time. Support staff such as housekeeping, transport and information, and others served on a number of floors. Additional personnel such as private duty nurses, nurses who were "floated" from other floors to pick up slack in staffing, and other staff also were often on the floor. In most cases, there was little regularity in the assignment or presence of staff who were not full-time members of the unit. Indeed, most people who performed work on the floor either were not permanently assigned to the unit or did not work there full-time (or even a majority of the time). This raised an important question: Where did the unit begin, and where did it end? And that led to other questions such as: To what extent could data on rotational staff job satisfacton be viewed as a valid reflection of events occurring on the unit?

2. *Shifting Consulting Strategy.* As the history of the project indicates, the consulting work differed from the preplanned activity originally envisioned. In practice, the consultants' work tended to be evolutionary. The first consulting group refused to articulate a plan of action and would not provide a set of predicted outcomes. The second group did provide a general plan of action, but, like the first, did not offer specific predicted outcomes. Also, the actual consulting activities tended to deviate somewhat from the planned activities. As a result, it was difficult to determine in advance what variables would be affected by the consultation—or even the location of consulting activities. This placed limits on the use of the measures originally constructed.

3. *Lack of Performance Measures.* The attempts to identify performance data consistent with the behavioral-economic measure guidelines quickly ran into problems. The first issue encountered was how to measure the effectiveness of a patient care unit. In areas where measures could be identified (such as absenteeism, overtime, unit costs, and so on), it was found that the hospital did not collect data on a patient care unit basis. So some data were not retrievable or were retrievable only through taking data by hand from individual employee records for each day of employment on the unit. This greatly limited the nature and quality of data available on unit performance and employee behavior.

4. *Contamination and Comparability of the Control Unit.* When the pilot surgical unit was originally chosen, another surgical unit was identified as a control unit. An implicit assumption was that the QWL project would probably expand to include as many as four or five experimental units and an equal number of comparable control units. But several factors made this approach unworkable. First, the project never expanded to other patient care units, so opportunities to generate additional control units did not occur. Second, because boundaries of and membership in patient care units were unclear, a relatively small population of full-time employees worked in each unit. Approximately twenty-five people were identified as full-time staff of each unit—an insufficient number for making adequate statistical comparisons. Finally, the control unit was in the same pavilion of the hospital as the experimental unit. (The control unit was on the second floor, while the experimental unit was on the fifth floor.) So as the consultant activities moved up the nursing hierarchy and began to focus on the assistant director of nursing (who had responsibility for the entire pavilion) and her team of nursing supervisors (including the supervisor for the control unit), the chances for contamination of the control unit grew. Therefore, the original strategy of a comparable unit for each experimental unit could not be implemented.

5. *Weak and Nonsupportive QWL Structure.* In theory, the quality of work life committees should provide support for measurement and data gathering. At Parkside, while the QWL steering committee did not place active roadblocks in the way of data collection, neither did it supply much help. While individual members did give general support for data collection (including letters from management to key supervisors and approval of union leaders for data collection), relatively little assistance was obtained in identifying additional sources of data or in dealing with resistance to data collection in the different

departments (accounting, medical records, and so on). Committee members showed relatively little interest in data collection and failed to show up when asked for questionnaire administrations.

Because the actual conditions at Parkside differed significantly from those assumed in the construction of the measurement package, many of the original instruments and procedures proved to be unworkable or unapplicable. First, the questionnaire lost some of its value. Because of the small number of full-time staff, any questionnaire data would have proven less useful than in cases where large units were available. Furthermore, problems occurred because many of the questions were not applicable to the situation. For example, the questionnaire asked for perceptions of the behavior of one's direct manager or supervisor. Parkside subjects were not sure who that person was. Was he or she the senior clinical nurse (head nurse) or the nursing supervisor? In either case, since there were changes between shifts, which particular person was being rated? In addition, much of the nurses' work was supervised by physicians. Were they to be considered in the questions? Similarly, many of the nursing aides and assistants were actually supervised by registered nurses. Were these individuals to be considered? Such problems of ambiguity existed with regard to a number of the questionnaire's sections.

Second, the behavioral-economic data guidelines simply could not be used. Data were unavailable, so standard methods for measuring and costing out absenteeism, turnover, and unit performance could not be employed.

Third, the general observational guidelines were inadequate for doing intensive observational work in a relatively complex environment. While they provided some basic principles, the lack of instruments, sampling plans, coding schemes, and the like presented major problems.

A New Assessment Strategy

In light of these above problems, the research team found that it had to develop a new measurement and assessment strategy. During the first six months of the project, it became apparent that the basic Michigan measurement package would be inadequate for describing and assessing the Parkside project. Therefore work began on a new approach more applicable to Parkside. The assessment strategy that evolved at Parkside had six major features. Each of these will be discussed individually.

First, the assessment strategy was still based on the concept of *multiple methods of data collection,* although the type and mix of methods were somewhat modified. Self-report data continued to be used although its role was downgraded. A shortened version of the Michigan questionnaire was employed, one which excluded many of the questions that (a) would not be affected by or related to the consultation work, and (b) would not be appropriate to a hospital patient care unit. The questionnaire is included in the Appendix. In addition, several new self-report instruments were developed, including an open-ended response format questionnaire that was used at the beginning of the project to gather background data on the unit and its relevant issues, a questionnaire on reactions to the training program on the unit, a questionnaire for use in survey feedback in the clinical services departments, and a post-project interview for use in debriefing key participants. In addition, informal unstructured interviews were conducted with staff as part of the ongoing observational work.

In addition to self-reports, a limited amount of data on behavior and performance was collected. In particular, absenteeism and overtime data for pilot unit personnel were obtained by copying the information directly from individual handwritten attendance records. Secondly, data from nursing audits—a highly structured, standardized observation method for measuring quality of nursing care—were assessed. These data sources and the methods of data collection and analysis will be discussed in the section on assessment of the pilot unit activities in Chapter 10.

The third basic data collection method was observation. The consultants decided to rely much more than originally planned on the observation of project-related events, activities, and behavior in the hospital. Observational methods provided the flexibility necessary for tracking the different components of the projects as they evolved. The specifics of the observational data collection will be discussed later.

Thus the assessment continued to rely on three major sources of data: self-reports, archival data, and observational data. The analysis strategy remained one of looking for convergence of results across methods as the basic means of assessing the validity of inferences.

The second major feature of the new assessment strategy was that it was *observation led.* The original intention was that the quantitative data provided by questionnaires and behavioral-economic data would provide the basic source for assessment of the project, and that observation would generate confirmational data. The observational work was seen as limited to infrequent, periodic visits to the site and the presence of an observer at major project events. Observation would thus provide somewhat richer data that could be used to explain the patterns and contributing factors underlying the primary assessment results from the more quantitative data sources. It would also provide the material for a narrative of the project.

At Parkside, this approach had to be reversed. Since the questionnaire and behavioral-economic measures could not be applied as planned, much less confidence could be placed in any results from them. The evolutionary consulting strategy made it difficult, as has been noted, to implement these more standardized data collection methods. In addition, the nature of the project at Parkside was turbulent, ambiguous, and unpredictable. Thus the research team felt that the most important data would be those which described how the project developed over time—including the ups and downs, the vicissitudes, and the dynamics of evolving and conflicting relationships between individuals and among groups. In many ways, the questionnaire and behavioral-economic measures could not have captured these phenomena, even if conditions had been right for comprehensive and rigorous use of these methods. The questionnaire is essentially a static measure; it produces self-reports of employee perceptions and attitudes at one point in time and thus may have inherent limitations as a means for generating useful descriptive data about dynamic processes. Behavioral-economic measures, while reflecting events over time in a more continuous manner, tend to focus on results of behavior, rather than the causal factors or the behavior itself.

Therefore observation was used as the project's primary method of data collection. Observational data would be employed to describe the events and arrive at initial judgments on the effects of the project and the consultation. The questionnaire and behavioral data would then be used to test the observation-developed hypotheses.

However, the team had relatively few guidelines for doing such observational work. The observational literature provided little direction aside from the two extreme options of unstructured participant observation and highly structured and focused laboratory-type observational instruments. (See Hanlon, 1980, for a review of the observational literature.) Therefore the team began to develop its own observational methodology.

The basic question in observation, as in any data collection method, is that of structure. As the data collection becomes more structured, it also becomes more standardized and thus more reliable and stable over time and location. On the other hand, standardization leads to a loss of flexibility and adaptiveness and thus to the potential loss of richness and ultimate data validity (Nadler, 1977).

In observation, there are basically two structuring decisions to be made. The first concerns the extent to which the actual watching of behavior should be structured by specifying the nature of events to be observed. The second concerns how much to structure the recording of the events being watched. Given the unpredictable and evolutionary nature of the project, the researchers believed that attempting to specify and structure what to watch would create the same problems for observation that were encountered in the application of the other data collection methods. Therefore they decided not to structure the content of observation except in the most general terms. All observers would have training in a general framework and would be given a set of variables for understanding organizational behavior (see Nadler & Tushman, 1977). But this was only to provide a general focus for observation and a common language for discussing and labelling the phenomena observed.

The major structuring decision involved the method for recording the observations and the coding of the recorded entries to facilitate later retrieval and analysis. First, a standard observational recording format was developed. For all observations, the observer was asked to record three types of information in separate locations. The first type was labelled *detailed observations*. They included the observed events, behaviors, activities and the like recorded in as factual, descriptive and noninterpretative a manner as possible. The ultimate test of objectivity was whether these data could be shown to those who were observed (they were not, in actuality) with little fear of giving offense. The second category was called *interpretations*. Here the observer listed his or her interpretation of the events, including statements of causality, identification of patterns, hypotheses about emotions and so on. The third category concerned the feelings of the observer in the situation. The assumption was that the separation of these three types of data would yield the richest yet most analyzable type of information.

The observations were also labelled according to two very general categories. The first concerned the physical (or organizational) setting in which the observation was made. A number of key physical and organizational locations were identified early in the project, and more were added later. For example, the pilot unit was one location, the control unit another, and the steering committee (regardless of where it physically met) a third. Within each location, a second label was attached, classifying the observation by the category of event that was observed. For example, in the pilot unit setting, events might include staff conferences or random observations of on-unit functioning. A completed sample observation form is included in the Appendix.

The final aspect of the observational methodology was a sampling plan. It required that all project activities be observed to the greatest degree possible. Thus observers should be present at all steering committee meetings, all consultant work, all project task force or group meetings, and so on. In addition, regular observations of the pilot unit at randomly sampled times would be made to provide data on life on the unit when the consultants were not present. This was seen as a way to generate observational data regarding the project's effects upon the ongoing functioning of the unit. (For further information on these observational data structuring methods, see Nadler, Perkins & Hanlon, 1983.)

Over the project's life, approximately 1500 observations were made concerning the project, the pilot unit, and the various subproject activities. They were then summarized by setting an events code to construct the project narrative and also to develop basic conclusions about the effects of the project on the organizational units involved.

The third major feature of the assessment strategy was the use of *add-on control* units. Given the inadequacy of the original control units, efforts were made to find useful and meaningful control units for different portions of the project. An example is the identification of controls for the pilot unit. The original design, as mentioned above, involved the identification of another surgical unit in the same pavilion as a comparable control unit. Therefore the first wave of questionnaire data (in late 1976 and early 1977) involved these two units. By late 1977, the problems with this approach had become clear. In addition, it appeared that the organizational mirroring subproject would be initiated and that data would also have to be collected from patient care units involved in this effort. Thus it was decided to identify additional units to serve as controls. Four other patient care units were identified. Two of them were randomly chosen from all of the hospital's medical and surgical units except those in the pavilion to which the original pilot and control units belonged. Two others were randomly chosen from the set of units that had been identified as the units to be included in the initial mirroring activities. Thus, by administration of the second questionnaire, the design had been altered to provide data from six different units. They were as follows:

One unit—the experimental unit (the pilot unit)
One unit—the original control unit
Two units—two random controls with no mirroring activity
Two units—two random controls with mirroring activity

As it turned out, the mirroring activity never reached the point where major effects were expected or observed on the units involved. As a result, the final design involved the experimental unit, the original control unit, and four randomly chosen controls. For assessment of the pilot unit consultation, questionnaire and behavioral data were obtained for all six units for the duration of the project.

The fourth feature of the assessment was the development of ad hoc measures. In other words, as the project evolved, new measures were developed as the situations permitted. The Michigan package envisioned a set of preplanned measurement tools to be applied in a preset and planned fashion. As already noted, the consultation work tended to be more evolutionary than planned. As the consultants identified or were presented with opportunities to do what they saw as constructive work, they seized upon these opportunities even if they had not been anticipated originally. Therefore the actual consultation described in the history differed considerably from the anticipated consultation, which was to focus exclusively on patient care units. At this point in the book, the opportunistic strategy of consultation is not being evaluated. Rather, we are noting it because of the issues it presented for assessment. It required the team to develop new measures for collecting data on new and unplanned aspects of the project after those project elements were already underway.

An example is the development of the assessment tools for the clinical services survey feedback project. This project started very quickly as a result of contacts between a member of the second consulting group and the director of the clinical services departments. It was not anticipated in the original project write-up or in the initial discussions that the consultants had with the steering committee or the research team. The problem was that a new project had begun with little time for preconsultation baseline measurement, with a questionnaire-based consultative intervention, and with no viable controls (since the project included all of the clinical services departments). Therefore the research team used the following approach:

1.   The researchers bargained with the consultants over the content of the questionnaire. The resulting survey feedback questionnaire included some items and scales from the researcher's questionnaire (as used in the six patient care units) and some from the questionnaire that the consultants wanted to use for survey feedback.

2.   The researchers arranged to do observations of the feedback project activities, including meetings with department management, feedback meetings, and so on.

3.   The researchers developed a self-report form (as a log book) for the feedback meeting facilitators to use to report their own activities and the nature of the feedback meetings. These were to be used as sources for descriptive data about the feedback processes, which were to be the basis for a priori predictions of changes in individual clinical department functioning as reflected in the second questionnaire.

Thus in this case the research team had to modify its approach, limit its data collection, and develop new data collection instruments to evaluate a consultation as it developed. This process was repeated several times during the project.

A fifth characteristic of the assessment was its *decreasing intensity*. By the end of 1977, our opinion was that the project would not have a major impact on Parkside. The activities on the pilot unit had become stalled, the survey feedback effort in clinical services was faltering, and the mirroring project was having trouble getting started. These developments had implications for the measurement activities and in particular for the observational data collection. First, there was less to observe. Steering committee meetings became less frequent, and little was occurring on the pilot unit. Individuals on the units being observed were becoming less cooperative because they associated the researchers with a project that had provided few tangible benefits. More and more frequently, people in the hospital began asking the observers what they were observing. Second, after several months of this decreased activity level, the researchers began to question the benefits of continued intensive observation. It appeared that no new data, insights, or information were being collected through the observational work. Thus a decision was made to greatly decrease the frequency of observation and in particular to reduce the number of random observations (not connected with any project activity) to a very low level. Every few weeks, there was a visit to the unit, observations were made, and a discussion was held with key informants about whether there had been any new developments.

Sixth and finally, the assessment work was, of necessity, *limited in scope*. In particular, not all project activities were measured to the same degree. Basically, the research team was excluded from observing those consultation activities measurable only through observation but where observation tended to be intrusive. Typically, such activities involved the (second) consulting team working one-on-one with a particular person, or with two or three people. The consultants claimed that a silent observer at these sessions would be inhibiting and would interfere with the development of an effective client-consultant relationship. Especially affected was the so-called "communications network," which was observed only to a limited extent; the one-on-one meetings with the assistant director of nursing for the experimental unit's pavilion, which were observed only intermittently; and the consultant's work with the director of nursing and her assistant directors, which was not observed at all.

The assessment effort was also limited by lack of cooperation, particularly in the last phases of the project. In particular, a hospital staff member was assigned to evaluate the effects of the mirroring project, and ideally this individual could have collaborated with the research team. In practice, no serious effort to assess mirroring was really launched by those involved, especially when the mirroring effort appeared to be faltering.

In summary, the research team developed its own strategy for the project. This strategy, involving the six features discussed here, was the one which guided the measurement work, especially during the final two years of the project.

UNRESOLVED ISSUES IN ASSESSMENT

The assessment strategy just described was developed in response to the problems of attempting to apply a research design and technology in a difficult environment. In many ways the new strategy, though limited, was adequate for achieving the basic goals of documenting the project, describing how it evolved, and assessing its impact on both individual and organizational outcomes. However, a number of issues remained unresolved and thus plagued the researchers throughout the effort. It is important to note these problems, since they may have influenced or biased the data and conclusions. By identifying the problems, we hope to enable the reader to make his or her own determination of the extent to which these problems are reflected in the researchers' final conclusions.

The first major unresolved issue concerned the role of the research team as a third party assessor. The quality of work life intervention design and the measurement package were designed for a research team in the role of a third party, with the first party being the site organization (including both labor and management), and the second being the consultants. The rationale was that the assessors would be objective observers of the events and would therefore have no vested interest in how the project turned out. (See Lawler, 1977, for a discussion of this approach.) It was assumed that the research team would be able to maintain this neutral third party role.

In reality, the third party role is difficult to maintain in any situation (see Nieva & Perkins, 1980), and Parkside presented particular difficulties. Early in the project, when the NQWC representative failed to develop adequate leadership for the steering committee, the researchers were often drawn into the leadership role. Individuals would direct questions at the researchers who were then faced with the choice of not answering (and thus threatening the very existence of the project and the viability of the researcher role) or answering and abandoning their neutral role. Each incident thus required a decision, and while neutrality was generally maintained, in some cases the researchers did get pulled into project activities.

The need for building rapport with subjects in order to get data led to problems. When the first consulting group began to perform poorly, individuals on the pilot unit approached one of the researchers. The people on the unit stated that they trusted the researchers but could not talk or communicate well with the consultants, that the researchers were present more often and thus seemed more interested in them than the consultants, and that they were looking to the researchers for help. The researchers referred the individuals to the NQWC representative who had initiated the project, but clearly, in the eyes of many, the researchers had been pulled out of the third party role. Another result was that the first consulting group viewed the researchers as adversaries.

An effort was made to develop a more collaborative relationship between the second consulting group and the researchers. It was facilitated by the fact that one of the researchers had worked with two of the consultants in past projects. Even so, at various times friction and conflict arose between the two groups because of their different priorities. The exclusion of the researchers from observation of certain activities mentioned above was symptomatic of the low level (yet ever present) tension that existed between the consultants and researchers.

A second major unresolved issue was that of the feelings of the researchers during the various project phases. Because of the researchers' involvement in multiple roles, because of the long involvement of key research team members (from two to three years), and because of the need to build relationships with individuals in the hospital, the members of the research team found it difficult to maintain a detached, uninvolved, and neutral stance.

Over time, the researchers experienced a variety of intense emotions. The initial feelings combined excitement on the one hand with frustration on the other—frustration regarding what was perceived as poor entry and start-up work by the NQWC representatives.

These feelings of frustration deepened and intensified during the consultant selection process because the researchers believed that a poor choice was being made but felt unable to exert any influence over the choice process.

As the first consulting group began to run into problems, the researchers frequently felt embarrassed at being associated with a project that was failing and was not being conducted effectively. This embarrassment created conflict when unit members approached the researchers about problems with the consultants. The latter were tempted to strongly support and identify with the unit members and thus distance themselves from the consultants. But they simply referred the individuals to the NQWC representative.

When the second consulting group began its work, feelings of excitement and hope for the project again developed, but these soon turned into frustration as this second group ran into problems in the nursing hierarchy and with the steering committee.

Finally, as the project began to move into a cyclical pattern of failure, the researchers experienced an extended period of depression.

The two problems, intergroup conflict and the intense emotions of the researchers, were not ones that could easily be dealt with by modifications of instruments, procedures, or research designs. Thus they persisted and remained basically unresolved throughout the course of the project and indeed through the process of data analysis and the writing of this report. It is difficult for us to assess how these issues affected the choice of data, the analytic procedures, and the interpretations made, but readers can take these factors into consideration as they review the results and discussion sections.

SUMMARY

The research team was charged with collecting data which would make possible the documentation, description, and assessment of the Parkside Quality of Work Life Project. Early in the project it became apparent that the research procedures and tools were not appropriate for the particular setting, so a new research strategy, centering on observational measures and ad hoc research designs, was developed. The result was a significantly different research design, but one which appeared to be more adequate for the task at hand. At the same time, the intense emotional reactions of observers involved with the same organization for three years raised issues about the viability of their third party role. These issues were not resolved and may have had an effect on the process and outcomes of the assessment activities.

CHAPTER TEN

Assessment of the Quality of Work Life Project

During its tenure at Parkside, the Evans consulting team shifted its focus of attention several times in searching for viable client groups within the hospital. We described the consultant's strategy and where it led them in Chapters 6 through 8. In this chapter, we present our formal evaluation of these different streams of consultant activity.

The consultants began by working on the pilot unit, Barnard 5. Frustration, lack of progress in scheduling changes, and a desire to make a hospitalwide impact led the consultants to other areas of the hospital. In the administrative hierarchy of the department of nursing, they began work on a subproject that became known as the Nursing Communication Network. They also started the Clinical Services Subproject. The latter diverged into two streams of activity—survey feedback and organizational mirroring. They also returned to the pilot unit in a renewed attempt to change floor behavior and obtain union involvement.

Our task as an evaluation team was to examine the activities of the consultants and assess the changes that occurred as a result of each subproject. In the process, we came into contact with various clients and dealt with a number of project goals, ranging from the broad "improving quality of work life" to the more narrow "improving conflict resolution skills."

The consultants' shifts of focus created problems for us. For example, when they were dealing with the nursing hierarchy, we became familiar with nursing units and quality patient care, the rivalries between nursing floors, and the conflicts between nurses, nursing aides, and doctors. Then the consultants shifted to another project, with a whole new cast of characters, in the clinical services division. Here administrators and doctors ran service activities. We suddenly had to orient ourselves to different people and different systems of working while trying to evaluate what was being done.

To establish a "fit" with project uncertainty, we developed an assessment strategy that had flexibility as its basic tenet. The original assessment strategy (see Chapter 9) was to attempt to clarify the goals of a particular project and to collect pretest and posttest questionnaire data to determine whether those goals were achieved. This strategy, however, was seldom easy to implement. Project goals shifted in midstream; control subjects transferred to experimental units; often, evaluation work had to be curtailed to avoid contamination of consultants activities.

For example, on the pilot unit, Barnard 5, we collected questionnaire data in late 1975 as a pretest for pilot unit project change. We chose as a control site Barnard 2, another surgical unit. It would not have been appropriate to do the posttest questionnaire for almost two years. But the turnover rate assured that after such a time lapse, the sample would be quite different from the original. Also, by then Barnard 2 could no longer be called a control since its administration had become part of the "experimental" nursing communication network. Finally, by that time the consultant team had changed, and a new set of pilot project goals had been developed. Other roadblocks to clean assessment arose because of the consultants' belief that we were an intrusion upon their one-on-one meetings. We didn't go to such meetings, which meant that no data were collected for some projects. Also, the bloodbank mirroring group decided to collect its own data. We didn't wish to interfere with the functioning of that group, so no data were collected by us. The result was uninterpretable numbers.

Flexibility was essential. We supplemented survey data collection with observation, the use of existing hospital data (henceforth called archival data), and interviews. Observation gave us a closer look at the people we were assessing and at the day-to-day behaviors that were the object of change. We learned what actually happened and what people expected from the project. Archival data provided information on sick hours and nursing performance and could serve as a means to compare project groups to a variety of controls. Finally, interviews provided subjective information on project activities, that is, the perceptions of the players, which can often be more important than "objective" reality. Multiple methods were used so that if one didn't provide the information we needed, another could. If two data sources led to conflicting conclusions, a third could be examined. (See Table 10.1 for a summary of projects and assessment methods and Table 10.2

Table 10.1.   Summary of Subprojects and Assessment Methods

Subproject	Assessment Methods
Pilot Unit	
Fall 1975–summer 1976 Preproject assessment, Wheaton Associates team hired and dismissed	Observation, preliminary interviews, first wave questionnaire, absenteeism
Fall 1976–fall 1977 Evans group activities—diagnostic work, staff conferences, resident orientation	Observation, absenteeism, first wave audit data
Fall 1977–spring 1978 Evans group activities—training program to improve unit member skills	Observation, absenteeism, training, program questionnaire.
Spring 1978–summer 1978 Evans group winds down activities and leaves	Observation, final interviews, second wave questionnaire, absenteeism, second wave audit data
Fall 1978–winter 1979 Follow-up data collection after all activity has ended	Observation, third wave questionnaire, third wave audit data
Nursing Department Communications Network	
Winter 1977–spring 1978	Observation, interviews
Clinical Services Survey Feedback	
Fall 1976–spring 1978	Observation, interviews, questionnaire, log books
Organization Mirroring	
Fall 1977–fall 1978	Observation

for a summary of data collection methods and a rationale for their use.)

This section is divided into four parts. The first reports on the pilot unit subproject. It deals with both the early phase of group problem-solving meetings and physician orientation and the late phase of training program activity. The second part discusses the nursing communication network, which represented the beginning of the consultants' "branching out" strategy that took them from the pilot unit to the pavilion and beyond. The third and fourth parts report on the two clinical services subprojects: survey feedback and organizational mirroring (the subproject aimed at improving linkages between nursing units and the clinical services division). Each part includes a short summary of subproject activities, the methodology used to assess change, results, and discussion.

Table 10.2. Summary of Assessment Methods and Rationale

Phase	Project Activities	Obs.	Int.	Quest.	Absent.	Audit.	Rationale
Preproject work							
Fall 1975	Unit staff chooses consulting group with steering committee. No on-site activity.	X	X	X	X		Pretest measures. These data represent baseline level attitudes and behaviors prior to consultant activity.
Wheaton Associates							
Winter 1976	Wheaton team begins diagnostic work.	X			X		Observation was used to keep track of what was taking place on unit. No projects were started so no changes were expected.
Spring 1976	Long consultant absences.	X			X		
Summer 1976	Wheaton team dismissed.	X					
Evans Team							
Fall 1976	Evans team begins diagnostic work.	X			X		The Evans group activities were constantly monitored via observation and absentee-ism data. A second questionnaire was administered in the fall of 1977 to assess the changes resulting from Evans group activities and in
Winter 1977	Staff conferences started.	X			X		
Spring 1977	Orientation for residents started. Low activity.	X			X	X	
Fall 1977	Training program for improved unit staff skills started.	X		X	X		

Winter–Spring Summer 1978	Consultants wind down activities and leave.	X		X	the winter of 1978 to assess the results of the training program. Nursing audit data became available which coincided with early and late consultant activity, hence an indication of behavioral changes on the part of nursing staff. Interviews in summer of 1978 recorded perceptions of project results.
Postproject Fall 1978– winter 1979	Unit functioning normally—no consultant activity.		X	X	Organizational change projects can have short-lived effects which die out or lagged effects which don't show up for several months. Observations, a third questionnaire administration, and audit data were used to assess changes in evidence up to six months following consultant activity.

THE BARNARD 5 PILOT UNIT SUBPROJECT

The QWL project on Barnard 5, the original pilot site of the Parkside Quality of Work Life Project, began in January of 1976 with the initial diagnostic work of the Wheaton Associates team and continued through the project's official termination in August of 1978. The Barnard 5 subproject was the only one that spanned the entire time frame of the Parkside project.

As indicated in the narrative, the level of activity on Barnard 5 fluctuated greatly throughout the project. For example, from April of 1976 until the dismissal of the Wheaton group the following August, there was virtually no QWL activity on the unit. For several months after the Evans team began its work in September of 1976, the involvement level of Barnard 5 employees increased greatly. But when Evans and Meyer realized that the project was not going to transcend the boundaries of a single nursing unit, they branched out and began to search for new clients in other parts of the hospital. This meant a reduction in the consulting resources devoted to Barnard 5.

As described in Chapter 9, the ebb and flow of the Parkside project meant significant and often rapid changes in our assessment strategy. From exclusive reliance upon questionnaire surveys and archival data within a specified amount of time, we gradually switched to more flexible methods such as participant observation and face-to-face interviews. So while beginning with a survey questionnaire designed specifically for measuring organizational change (including the types of changes resulting from QWL projects), we also came to rely on archival data, interviews, and participant observation.

Questionnaire Data

The attitudes and perceptions of Barnard 5 staff were measured at three different points during the project. In late 1975, questionnaires were administered to the staff on Barnard 5 and the staff on a matched control unit, Barnard 2. The latter was another surgical floor within Barnard Pavilion, one which hospital management and the unions felt was comparable to the pilot unit in terms of physical layout, staffing, and types of patients served. The questionnaire was a modified version of the Michigan Organizational Assessment Questionnaire (Seashore, Lawler, Mirvis & Cammann, 1983), which is described in Chapter 9. From the 183 items on the original questionnaire, we selected those modules and scales that were appropriate to the Parkside project. We also changed the wording of the questionnaire to make it suitable for administration to employees of a tertiary care hospital such as Parkside.

The questionnaire was readministered in November and December of 1977. By then it was apparent that the original control unit, Barnard 2, was not an unbiased control. At that time, Evans' consulting work with the nursing administrative hierarchy in Barnard Pavilion could have been regarded as having had an impact on Barnard 2 as well as on the experimental unit, Barnard 5. To mitigate this contamination, we randomly selected additional control units from a list of all medical-surgical units in the hospital.

Altogether, six units were included in the second questionnaire administration: Barnard 5, Barnard 2, and the four random control units (total $N = 96$). Finally, in January of 1979, five months after the termination of the quality of work life project, the questionnaire was readministered to the six units included in the modified design. Technically, our research was a pretest, posttest control group design (Campbell & Stanley, 1963). It could be diagrammed as such:

X	O	X	experimental unit	(Barnard 5)
X	O	X	control unit	(Barnard 2)

The basic issue tested by our questionnaire research design was whether employee attitudes on Barnard 5 had changed as a result of consultant and project activity.

Factor analysis, using the Varimax orthogonal rotation procedure, was carried out on the modules of the Michigan Organizational Assessment Questionnaire scales in order to verify the instrument's intended scale structure and to compute scales. The factor analysis showed that the intended scale structure closely described item patterns from the six unit data. The resulting scales and their coefficients of reliability (Cronbach's coefficient α, see Nunnally, 1978) were as follows:

Scale Name	Coefficient α
Satisfaction With Achievement	.77
Satisfaction With Co-Workers	.91
Chance to Accomplish Things	.89
Satisfaction With Extrinsic Rewards (for example pay, fringe benefits)	.69
Trust and Involvement With Co-Workers	.75
Work Group Conflict	.78
Freedom on the Job	.74
Satisfaction With Patient Care	.80

The project steering committee did not establish specific goals or objectives for the Barnard 5 project. The organizational development plan submitted by the consultants on October 12, 1976 was general in nature, but it did specify two major objectives:

1. Develop health care improvement teams on Barnard 5 to plan and implement organizational development strategies.
2. Train individual team members to use applied behavioral science skills and techniques throughout the Parkside system. Focus on increasing skills in problem solving, communications, supervision, group decision making, and conflict resolution.

In the absence of objectives regarding specific changes in employee behavior on the pilot unit, we reviewed written output of the consultant group and observational data to generate change hypotheses. Table 10.3 reports the changes expected of a successful project for each of the scales and presents the rationale for each prediction. Basically, we hypothesized that there would be major improvements regarding relations between co-workers, work group conflicts, and the chance to accomplish things. There would be small improvements in satisfaction with patient care, achievement and freedom on the job. Finally, there would be no change in satisfaction with extrinsic rewards or control over firing and promoting people.

Table 10.4 reports the means and differences in means between the pilot and control units, for both the second and third waves of data collection. Wave 1 results were not used in this analysis because turnover had resulted in a significantly different pilot unit population, and Barnard 2 unit was no longer an isolated control unit. Therefore Wave 2 can be viewed as only a posttest design reflecting the difference between the pilot and control units following the initiation of staff conferences and resident orientations.

Of the seven scales predicted to indicate major or minor positive changes, only the satisfaction with achievement scale showed a significant difference between the pilot and control units. But the difference was negative, indicating significantly less satisfaction with achievement on the pilot unit. All other difference measures were not significant, although each scale measuring interaction with co-workers (satisfaction with co-workers, trust and involvement with co-workers, and work group conflicts) indicated that the pilot unit was more negative than the control units. Individual level outcomes (chance to accomplish things and satisfaction with patient care), however, were more positive for the pilot unit.

Wave 3 data were collected in the fall of 1979, when the entire project, including the Barnard training program, had been completed. In comparing the differences between the pilot and control units at T2 to the differences at T3, no clear patterns emerged. The pilot unit exhibited positive changes compared to the control units in three predicted areas: satisfaction with achievement, satisfaction with co-workers, and handling work group conflicts. But only in work group conflicts was there a major gain over the control unit. As predicted, no change occurred in satisfaction with extrinsic rewards. Nor was there change in satisfaction with patient care, which meant the pilot unit was still more positive than the control units, though not significantly so. In all other areas—chance to accomplish things, trust and involvement with co-workers, freedom on the job, and control over promoting and firing people—the pilot unit was becoming more negative relative to the control units, even in areas where major changes in a positive direction were predicted. Apparently, the pilot unit employees became more cognizant than the control unit employees of the limits to their power to accomplish things in the organization. Yet the former also seemingly became better able than the latter to manage work group conflicts.

Archival Data

Two sets of archival data proved useful in evaluating the impact of the QWL project. The first was the pay records kept by Parkside for all employees. We used these records to gather data on employee absenteeism before, during, and after the QWL project. The objective was to determine if the Barnard 5 project reduced absenteeism on the floor relative to absenteeism on other comparable nursing units in the hospital. Previous research showed absenteeism to be a behavioral measure closely related to job satisfaction (Vroom, 1964). The costs of absenteeism include over-staffing and increasing the reliance on inexperienced employees (Nadler, Hackman, & Lawler, 1979).

The specific hypothesis tested here was that the quality of work life project activities on Barnard 5 had a significant effect on employee absenteeism; specifically, that absenteeism would be lower on the pilot unit than on comparable units with no QWL activity.

The second set of useful data was a study on nursing performance and care undertaken by the research division of the Parkside department of nursing. This study coincided in time with the QWL project. We were able to obtain these data from the department of nursing and carried out a secondary analysis of them to discover if the Barnard 5 project led to improvements in nursing performance on the unit relative to other comparable units in the hospital.

Table 10.3. Predicted Change on Pilot Unit Questionnaire Measures

Change Indicator	Predicted Change	Rationale for Prediction
Scale 1		
Satisfaction with achievement	Small improvement	Intrinsic satisfaction, for example, "Doing my job well gives me a good feeling" was not an articulated objective of the project. One would expect some improvement since job satisfaction is related to more specific areas of project-related change.
Scale 2		
Satisfaction with co-workers	Major improvement	Much of the consultants' work on the pilot unit was directed at improving relations among unit staff. The staff conferences, the training program for unit staff, the physicians orientation, and the leadership training provided at the supervisory and administrative levels were all directed toward this goal.
Scale 3		
Chance to accomplish things	Major improvement	One of the often most stated goals of the projects was to "give everyone a say." The staff conferences and the training program were intended to provide staff, particularly lower level staff, with a sense that they could suggest changes and act on these changes.
Scale 4		
Satisfaction with extrinsic rewards	No improvement	The areas of pay and fringe benefits were never defined as objects of concern within the project.

Scale 5 Trust and involvement with Co-workers	Major improvement	Improving communication among staff was one of the most strongly articulated goals of the consultant group. Improvement in communications and common involvement in project activities could be expected to lead to positive change in trust and involvement among staff.
Scale 6 Work group conflicts	Major improvement	The training program, doctors orientation, leadership training and staff conferences were all seen as vehicles for reducing work group conflicts. This was one of the major goals of the project.
Scale 7 Freedom on the Job	Small improvement	The articulated goal of giving staff more say in how to do their work was never really given much emphasis in project activities. Still, one would expect some spillover from problem-solving meetings.
Scale 8 How much say in promoting and firing people	No improvement	Control over promotion, firing, and hiring were never viewed as the province of the quality of work life project.
Scale 9 Satisfaction with patient care	Small improvement	Presumably with increased meetings and planning, the unit would be working on ways to improve patient care.

Table 10.4.   Scale Means and Mean Differences for the Pilot and Control Units for Two Waves of Questionnaire Administration

	Wave 2—Fall 1977			Wave 3—Winter 1979		
	Pilot	Control	Difference	Pilot	Control	Difference
Satisfaction with achievement	5.71	6.25	−.54*	5.97	6.09	−.12
Satisfaction with Co-workers	4.83	5.23	−.40	5.17	5.42	−.25
Chance to accomplish things	5.12	4.79	.34	4.63	5.34	−.71
Satisfaction with extrinsic rewards	4.62	4.77	−.15	4.90	5.01	−.11
Trust and involvement with Co-workers	4.82	4.85	−.03	4.83	5.02	−.19
Work group conflicts	3.89	4.04	−.15	4.22	3.74	.49
Freedom on the job	3.97	4.24	−.27	3.47	4.10	−.63
How much say in promoting and firing people	1.95	1.66	.29	1.33	1.78	−.45
Satisfaction with patient care	3.54	5.41	.13	3.20	3.08	.12

*Note. $p < .05$.
1-7 scale with 7 indicated most positive response.

Absenteeism. Information on total hours worked, total sick hours, supervisor sick hours, unit clerk sick hours, and overtime hours per unit per week was collected for eleven quarters spanning the length of the project. (We are measuring absenteeism here as sick hours and overtime hours on the unit.)

The percentage of total sick hours was calculated by dividing the total sick hours by the total number of hours worked per week. Then the percentage for the quarter was calculated, and paired t-tests were run to determine if there were significant differences between the pilot unit and the controls.

Figure 10.1 records the differences between the percentage of total sick hours for the pilot and control units for each quarter. Two quarters showed significant differences, with the pilot unit exhibiting an increase in total sick hours near the end of 1977 and the beginning of 1978. There were no other significant differences between the pilot and control units for any other quarters with respect to total sick hours, supervisory sick hours, or unit clerk sick hours. As for overtime hours, the percentage for the pilot unit fell significantly below the control units for one quarter at the end of 1977.

Project activities accounted for only a small percentage of unit absenteeism. However, there was an increase in total sick hours during a period of intense consultant activity (training programs, staff conferences, resident orientation, windup activity). This may have contributed slightly to the low attendance at the training sessions. It was more indicative, however, of a lack of enthusiasm of some unit employees for project activities. The unit was able to achieve low overtime for one quarter, but otherwise did not achieve low levels of absenteeism compared to the control units.

Audit Data.   During the evaluation of change on the experimental unit, we discovered that the nursing administration in conjunction with the Healthtech consulting group was conducting a hospitalwide nursing audit. This audit was a framework for monitoring the quality of nursing care. More specifically, the audit used at Parkside (developed by Medicus Systems Corporation in cooperation with two of its clients, the Rush-Presbyterian-St. Luke's Medical Center in Chicago and the Baptist Medical Center in Birmingham, Alabama, and funded by the Division of Nursing of the Bureau of Health Resources Development, Department of Health, Education & Welfare) rated direct patient care as well as management and support services on nursing units (Hegyvary & Haussman, 1976). Since the timing of the audit corresponded to critical points in the Parkside project, we decided to use the data to monitor change on the pilot unit.

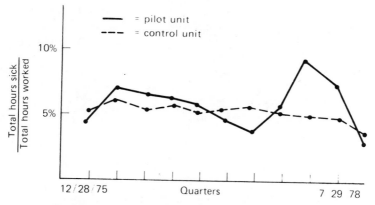

Figure 10.1.   Differences between the pilot and control units on percentage of total sick hours per quarter.

Our interest in these data stemmed from the finding of the Medicus group that:

> In many instances it was possible to link changes in quality [of nursing] with particular happenings on the unit in question (i.e., inadequate supervision), or in the hospital as a whole (i.e., low staff morale because of loss of personnel to a competing institution).

Previous research carried out by Medicus Systems Corporation indicated that nursing units with higher audit scores were structurally distinct and had more favorable staff attitudes, better reported quality of leadership, and more job satisfaction (Jelinek et al., 1974). This was consistent with the findings of the Georgopolos and Mann (1962) study of community general hospitals, which suggested that the quality of nursing care may be more susceptible to organizational influences than the quality of medical care (Haussmann et al., 1978). Georgopolos and Mann's research also indicated that quality of nursing care is perhaps the most important factor in determining quality of patient care.

The Medicus group developed a model of the patient care system from its findings. (See Figure 10.2.) The model suggested that five interrelating variables (unit organizational structure, nursing leadership style, unit staff attitudes, supervisory staff attitudes, and nursing staff education) affect nursing performance. Since the QWL project was attempting to improve the first four of those variables to a greater or lesser degree, the extent of its impact ought to have been reflected in the audit data measuring nursing performance. Therefore this section will compare the audit for the periods before, during, and after the Evans consulting work.

The audit evaluated direct patient care by looking at the nursing process, defined as the "comprehensive set of nursing activities performed in the delivery of a patient's care" (Haussmann, 1978 p. 6). This process consisted of four phases: assessment of patient needs, planning

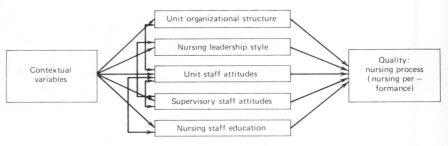

Figure 10.2.   Unit organizational structure.

for care, implementing the plan of care, and evaluating and updating the plan. The needs considered in the audit included both basic biological needs and such "higher order" needs as emotional support. With quality patient care also dependent on support services, these were monitored as well.

Nursing quality was monitored via a review of 10 percent of one month's patient census. The patients were randomly selected, with the limitation that 60 percent of observations be on the day shift and 40 percent on evenings. Each observation lasted about two and a half hours. After selection of a patient, he or she was classified according to severity of illness. Then the form containing the appropriate subset of the 256 criteria to observe and measure was filled out. (Appropriate patient needs were defined by severity of illnesses.) The unit was rated on both patient-specific and unit-specific criteria.

At the end of the audit, each unit had been rated on six objectives and twenty-eight subobjectives. The former were:

1. The plan of nursing care is formulated
2. The physical needs of the patient are attended
3. The nonphysical (psychological, emotional, mental, social) needs of the patient are attended
4. Achievement of nursing care objectives is evaluated
5. Unit procedures are followed for the protection of all patients
6. The delivery of nursing care is facilitated by administrative and managerial services

In January of 1977, the nursing audit was introduced by Healthtech and the nursing administration to thirty-three nursing units at Parkside. The problems of reliability and observer bias were approached in multiple ways. All observers were Parkside registered nurses, who reported either to the associate director of in-service education or the assistant director of nursing research. Thus the observers were knowledgeable about nursing care, but they were not connected with the specific units being measured. They received orientation and training regarding the instrument and were subjected to reliability testing. Interobserver reliability had to reach a minimum of 85 percent before administration of the audit could begin.

The first audit was completed in March of 1977. It corresponded to the period before the QWL project activities had expanded beyond the initial experimental unit, Barnard 5. The second audit was carried out during the first three months of 1978. By March of 1978, the consultants had completed the major part of their experimental unit intervention. Therefore the first time period (the interval from the first to the second audit) reflected the impact of the consultants' work on that unit. The third and last audit was carried out from September to November of 1978. Consultant activity had ended during the summer of 1978, bringing to a close the QWL project at Parkside. Therefore the second period (the interval from the second to the third audit) reflected any lasting impact of the project, as well as an increase in staffing during the summer and early fall of 1978.

If the project were successful, it was predicted that the experimental unit would experience a greater increase in nursing performance for the time period between the first two audits (T1 and T2) than the control unit and the rest of Barnard Pavilion. The performance gain would either increase or at least not erode between the second and third audits (T2 and T3) if the change were lasting. Table 10.5 compares the change in nursing performance between the pilot unit, the control units, and Barnard Pavilion. Since insufficient data were available for a parametric test, the nonparametric sign test was used to assess the significance of differences in change. More specifically, the null hypothesis of equal changes over time for the pilot and control units versus the alternative hypothesis of a larger change in nursing performance for the pilot unit was tested.

Table 10.5.   Comparison of Change in Nursing Performance Between the Pilot Unit, the Control Unit, and the Surgical Pavilion

Unit	Time Period	Number of Positive Changes in Performance
Pilot—Control	T1 to T3	19/26[a, b]
Pilot—Pavilion	T1 to T3	17/27
Pilot—Control	T1 to T2	12/28
Pilot—Pavilion	T1 to T2	11/28
Pilot—Control	T2 to T3	19/27[a]
Pilot—Pavilion	T2 to T3	19/28

Notes.
[a]$p < .05$ reject null hypothesis.
[b]The table is read as follows: when you subtract the change on each indicator of nursing performance between T1 and T3 on the control unit, from the change on each on the pilot unit, the difference is positive in 19 cases, negative in 7 cases, and 0 in 2 cases. Using the normal distribution to approximate the binomial value for $N = 26$, $P = .5$, and $\alpha = .05$, it can be seen that if 17 or more successes occur for 26 trials, the null hypothesis of equal change can be rejected.

Table 10.5 indicates that the pilot unit did not show significantly more improvement than either the control unit or Barnard Pavilion as a whole from T1 to T2. However, nursing performance did improve significantly for the pilot unit from T2 to T3. The pilot unit did finally experience significant increases for the entire time period T1 to T3, but the timing of the change was not as predicted. The change occurred after rather than during consultant activity. This indicates either that there was a lag effect in which change occurred only after the intervention was over or that the change was due to other factors. During the latter period (from T2 to T3), staffing on the floor was finally increased due to a different hospital project. It is possible that the nurses could not fully utilize their new skills nor implement floor meeting ideas until the increased staffing was achieved. Many nurses complained that because of understaffing, they did not have enough time to engage in project activities. Once new nurses arrived, those ideas might have been followed up. An alternative explanation is that the increase in staffing itself or the quality of the new nurses accounted for the increased performance. The experimental unit staff had become very sensitized to their poor staffing situation. Thus when staffing was improved in the second time period, it had a bigger impact on the experimental unit. Finally, interview data indicated that Barnard 5 got more and earlier additional staffing than the control units. This made it difficult to determine the extent of the QWL project's influence on increased audit scores as compared to the impact of the new staffing.

Interviews and Observation

At the beginning and end of the project, we conducted interviews with a stratified random sample of unit staff and members of the steering committee. The interviews involved structured questions but allowed for open-ended answers. The initial interview was primarily to familiarize us with the nature of the unit, the modes of operation, and the problems as perceived by staff. The final interview focused on perceptions of the project, its major activities, and its effects on life on the unit. Our goal was to have a record of staff perceptions to contrast with the more objective external ratings of change on the unit. Some individuals had been involved in the project for almost four years, and we wanted to know how they thought and felt about it.

The primary assessment data collection method of the Barnard 5 subproject was observation. Given the dynamic, continuous, and unpredictable nature of project activities, we felt that there could be no substitute for on-site observers who systematically watched the unit and the project activities. A semistructured observation approach was developed. Called *structured naturalistic observation,* it focused the observer's attention in a general way by providing key variables, while very specifically structuring how the observer would record and code observations of behavior sequences. (For a detailed description of this method, see Nadler, Perkins, & Hanlon, 1983.) The general sampling plan was to observe all project-related events. In addition, during the first two years of the project, observers performed intensive observations, which involved an observer being present on the unit for eighteen continuous hours so as to observe three different shifts at work.

Interviews. The semistructured interviews conducted at the end of the consultant intervention asked respondents to recall the project's chronology of events as well as their initial attitudes toward the project.

Initially, most participants were optimistic about the project. The following comments are illustrative:

Great need for such a project ...

For one thing I liked the idea that a lot of attention was going to be put on the floor ... That would be helpful to improve things.

People certainly did have reservations, but most felt like the interviewee who said she:

"approached it with an open mind and a lot of curiosity ... "

Two interviewees reported overtly skeptical initial attitudes:

the major feeling was that it was a managerial gimmick, aimed at getting things they couldn't get contractually ...

I couldn't figure out for the life of me why Big Brother suddenly became interested in the folks being unhappy.

Content analysis of the interview responses was performed to determine the themes most often expressed. The goals of the project mentioned by the interviewees were counted and sorted into categories, as were the final evaluations of project change.

Four goals were mentioned by at least three of those interviewed. Those mentioned most often were (1) improving patient care and (2) breaking down the barriers between workers at different hierarchical levels and between the different professional groups in order to bring hostility into the open and thus ultimately to promote better communication. Also mentioned by most interviewees was the goal of getting union and management to cooperate.

Almost all of the interviewees agreed that the QWL project produced some positive results while it was functioning. The effects seen by at least four of the twelve persons included: bringing floor problems into the open, that is, making it easier for the floor members to talk to one another; training individuals in problem-solving techniques; establishing a residents' orientation; creating a sense of pride on the floor; and producing better working relationships among the nursing staff. Further elaboration on the positive changes follows:

> Due to the project, we [the nurses and nursing aides] had an easier time talking to each other and expressing things. They weren't always very nice things, a lot of times they were bitter, such as 'you don't do your work' and 'you push work off on us.' But I think that what happened was that a lot of these things were expressed among nurses or nursing aides . . . . It made people feel easy about saying these things to each other . . . not only speaking amongst our own group.

> The project resulted in a little more understanding between the different groups that interact and interface on the floor, the nurses, nursing aides, between a supervisor and the staff people. There is a general understanding that each of us has our own problems . . . I think we understand a little bit more about what problems each of us face in our job—everybody has frustrations, things we would like to do that we can't do.

> There's a change with the safety reports. It is always replete with incidents of porters and maids getting stuck by needles which were not disposed of in the proper fashion. This dropped dramatically on the pilot unit.

> It was stressed in meetings that everyone should say something without fear of reprisal, recrimination . . . and after a while it started to happen.

The changes brought about by the project clearly were limited in many ways, as reported in the final interviews. One of the limitations mentioned by most individuals was that the project primarily benefited the nurses. Nursing aides and other nonprofessional employees were less affected. Doctors did not take part in most project activities, so change for them was obviously limited. Another limitation was that staffing problems deprived certain people of the time for participation. People indicated that:

> I think the nurses benefited. I'm not really sure about the nursing aides.

> I think there was an impact on certain individuals. Some of the nurses really developed a sense of the ways in which to involve other staff members in their work. I would say, however, that contrary to the initial goals of the project for the Hospital Workers' Union worker, who is not a nurse, work has not changed. That has not changed and that's too bad.

> The orientation has been a definite improvement on the floor. The nursing staff makes a big effort. The residents, on the other hand, acquiesce. They don't appreciate how the nursing service impacts on them.

> Attendance in the training program has been a problem. It is difficult to get nonprofessional people to the meetings . . . .

> Not enough time or staff.

Another difficulty in bringing about changes was people's skepticism about the permanence of these changes. A number of individuals pointed out that change was limited to a few persons, and that due to the high turnover, these would soon leave.

> I would say that overall I think the accomplishments were there but rather minimal, and I think that the major problem as I see it is that what accomplishments were achieved occurred during the time that the project was at its most active, and I concede that very quickly all those benefits will dissipate and be lost . . . because of the nature of the personnel up on the floor and the fact that now I think that the stability would be with people like Nancy Marullo and myself and so on. I must admit that in the last few months as I was negotiating to leave Parkside. . . .

> Whether it's going to continue when everybody that was involved in the project is off the floor, because that's eventually going to happen, I'm not sure . . . .

The final limitation stressed by the interviewees was that while attitudes had changed, behavioral change was not as forthcoming. Staff members also found it difficult to isolate what effects were attributable to the QWL project as opposed to external forces or to one or more of the fourteen other nursing projects in operation at the time of the QWL project.

> I would have really liked to see more programs, ongoing programs come out of it. Some of the things we've talked about—a library for staff, a patients' library, patient teaching conferences—things like that . . . the kind of concrete things that I think we are lacking.

Observation. The observational data confirmed most of what was said in the interviews about the project's effects. Some individuals profited greatly from the project. Nurses developed better ways of working together, and several individuals improved their leadership skills. The floor members had more of a sense of pride in their floor. There were also concrete changes—the residents' orientation and the staff conferences. But people would have liked to develop longer lasting, institutionalized programs. Instead, progress was impeded by staff turnover and an inability to get all groups involved in the project.

Table 10.6.   Training Program Questionnaire Means

To What Extent . . .	$\overline{\text{X}}$
1. Did participants in the training program learn to function as a group?	5.5
2. Did you enjoy participation in the training program?	6.7
3. Did the trainers provide useful information?	6.4
4. Did the trainers provide leadership when it was needed?	6.2
5. Did the trainers make the purpose of the sessions clear?	6.5
6. Overall, how would you rate the effectiveness of the trainers?	6.1

Note. For all questions, the scale range was one to seven, with the latter indicating the more favorable response.

The Training Program

In an attempt to bring the Hospital Workers' Union back into the project (see Chapter 7), the consultants developed a training program in interpersonal skills (group dynamics, conflict resolution, problem solving, and so on). It was originally designed solely for nonprofessional employees, but it grew to include other staff from Barnard 5 and a few from other floors in Barnard Pavilion. It began on a biweekly basis in December of 1977 and ran through the spring of 1978.

We assumed that change due to the training program would be picked up by the final attitude questionnaire, interviews, observation, audits, and absenteeism data. Nevertheless, another questionnaire was distributed following the training program. This was done because the consultant team member who ran the training program wanted evaluation data to use as feedback to unit employees. The questionnaire, developed by us for the consultant, included both fixed response and open-ended questions. Although not explicitly developed as an assessment instrument, the questionnaire data did provide an indication of employee attitudes about the program. Thus the responses are reported here.

Overall, the twelve participants who completed questionnaires were positive about the value of the sessions. As indicated in Table 10.6, the mean scores for the six close-ended questions were favorable. Responses to the open-ended questions were also generally positive. When asked to comment on the impact of the training on day-to-day relationships, participants gave the following responses:

I realized where the breakdown in communications is.

I have learned to take discussions objectively.

> I am very aware of others' feelings as I am conscious of my feelings.

> We relate to each other better.

> I have been able to look at situations from a different point of view and use some of the techniques practiced in the training session to affect a better working relationship.

> Better understanding of other staff members. Improved problem solving.

> We seem to have mutual understanding of what we want. It is almost an unspoken understanding for improvement within the unit. We are better able to reach agreement in problem solving and working together is more pleasurable.

> I've come to see the staff members in a multidimensional way, i.e., I have come to know them in other than their one role and have therefore felt closer to them as we have met twice monthly to share ideas and information.

> Attempting to apply the training methods to problems on the unit.

> It has given me a new outlook of self-development and dealing with others on different levels.

The responses indicated improvements in self-development and in understanding others' perspectives and needs. Not all responses were positive, and the negative answers indicated a phenomenon that also surfaced in the other pilot unit activities—a heightened awareness resulting from the intervention of what was wrong and could not be fixed quickly:

> No change.

> Adversely—it became increasingly clear that there was a breakdown in communication from supervisor to staff—little follow through—and need for assistant director to develop a different style.

Apart from the "after only" questionnaire administration, there were no attempts to measure explicitly the outcome of the training program. Interview, observational, and archival data were the sole sources of information on change over time.

In sum, the questionnaire data appeared to show that training program participants had a positive sense of accomplishment. But these data could not be used to evaluate broader unit change.

Discussion

The questionnaires, archival data, interviews, and observations all appeared to indicate that the project on the pilot unit was successful only to a small degree. During the course of the project, the unit did improve communication on the floor and increase its problem-solving capabilities. People felt more pride in their floor and learned some interpersonal skills during the course of the training sessions. In addition, nursing performance, as measured by the audit data, improved over the course of the project. Work group conflicts also appeared to have become less of a problem on the pilot unit than on the controls.

However, the project failed to achieve many of its initially stated goals. The attempt to get union and management and all levels on the floor working together did not get far. The project was primarily a nursing project—leaving the hospital workers and doctors out. Also, as one pilot unit member said: "We all come from such different backgrounds, countries and educations. Understanding each other is a tremendous problem." The project did little to break down these barriers. Furthermore, there was little change in membership behavior (absenteeism). The belief that all changes would be short-lived—disappearing as involved people left the floor—pervaded most people's thinking. With a 23 percent annual turnover rate, the changes were not expected to last long.

The changes that did last were a general feeling of goodwill and pride among the "veteran" staff members, improved communication and problem solving, and some increases in performance.

Increased goodwill appears to have resulted from increased interaction during the project; increased attention to the unit in general by outsiders, hospital management, and the like; and the accomplishments of the doctors' orientation and staff meetings. The training program resulted in increased sensitivity to others on the unit and improved problem-solving skills. The increased goodwill, however, appears to have been unrelated to ongoing patterns of behavior; it remained limited to those present during the project and confined to the nursing staff. Furthermore, there was a shared opinion that in the future—when the doctors' orientation would become more sporadic, the staff conferences would cease to be problem-solving arenas for all levels of staff, and the individuals involved in the project would leave the unit—these improved feelings and interactions would cease. Nevertheless, the individual skills that were developed would remain and could be used in other areas of the hospital.

The improved performance outcomes would have been concrete evidence of project success had their origin been clear. As is often true in evaluation research in field settings (Seashore, Lawler, Mirvis, & Cammann, 1983), it was not always possible to control another event coinciding with an intervention. This other event became an alternative hypothesis explaining the data results. Thus the change in the audit scores might have been the result of improved staffing resulting from a study by the top management of the nursing department aided by some external consultants and unrelated to the QWL project activities. The additional staff, the QWL project, or the two combined could have been responsible for the improved audit scores.

THE NURSING DEPARTMENT COMMUNICATION NETWORK SUBPROJECT

Introduction

In Chapters 6 through 8 we described the consultants' work with Nancy Marullo, the assistant director of nursing for Barnard Pavilion, and Merideth Klein, Parkside's director of nursing. This consulting activity began in June of 1977 and ended shortly before the project's termination in the following year. Most of the consultants' time was spent with Marullo and her supervisory staff, and since Evans and Meyer's objective was to improve the flow of communication within the Barnard nursing hierarchy, the project was labelled the "Barnard Communication Network." When Klein was included, it became the "Nursing Department Communication Network."

This set of activities is more difficult to describe than the other projects because it did not involve an easily derived and bounded target group, as did the Barnard 5 project, nor any standing committees to monitor and coordinate the activities. None of the unions were included; it was a "straight" management consulting project to expand the power base of and build legitimacy for the larger QWL project. Based on our observational records, we estimate that approximately one third of total consultant time was devoted to the communication network subproject.

Methods

Given the diffuse nature of this project, monitoring activities and establishing measurement objectives proved extremely difficult. It is important to note that this was the only sphere of project activity in which the consultants limited the presence of the Columbia research team. On a number of occasions, Bill Evans requested that research team members not attend one-on-one meetings, particularly meetings with Merideth Klein, on the grounds that an outsider's presence might be intrusive. The research team complied with all such requests. However, most consultant meetings with nursing department staff *were* open to members of the Columbia team. These included management training meetings for the assistant directors of nursing at Parkside and numerous meetings with the assistant director of nursing for Barnard Pavilion and various members of her supervisory staff.

Because of the project's nature and Evans and Meyer's concerns over the Columbia team's presence, measurement was limited to participant observation and extensive, open-ended interviews with Marullo and Klein at several points during the course of the QWL project.

Results

Evaluating the results of this area of Parkside activity is all but impossible, since objectives were never operationalized in a way to make them amenable to systematic analysis.

After the termination of the QWL project, Marullo and Klein were asked to evaluate the performance and helpfulness of the consultants. Klein gave them high marks overall, but she did not provide many specific examples of improvements that could be linked to the consultants or to the quality of work life project. Marullo offered a more mixed assessment. She concluded that the consultants, and especially Meyer, were helpful in a number of areas, including the clarification of the clinical supervisor's role. She felt that her management skills had improved as a result of the intervention. But she also believed that her involvement in the QWL project had been extremely time-consuming and probably not worth the effort.

The final interviews with Barnard 5 employees indicated that unit personnel noticed some differences in supervisory behavior. Specifically, they felt the clinical supervisor and assistant director of nursing for the Barnard Pavilion had gained leadership skills.

One nurse on the unit noted that:

> The consultants saw immediately that people like the assistant director, Mrs. Marullo, and the supervisors were not involved enough in the project. I think this changed. It was important to train these people, including the senior clinical nurses, in what it means to be a leader, in how to get things done. In my mind, that was a *very* important activity, and I think a lot of people benefited from that.

Overall, the communication network subproject did improve the quality of communication between supervisor levels and staff, although these improvements were not subject to any rigorous measurement strategy. It seems clear, however, that Evans and Meyer failed to implement the key strategy item on their "hidden agenda": to use the communication network project as a means of building the credibility of the Parkside Quality of Work Life Project.

Finally, despite their efforts, Evans and Meyer were never involved centrally in the larger nursing department reorganization plan. As we indicated in Chapters 8 and 9, much of the consultants' work was peripheral to senior management concerns.

CLINICAL SERVICES DEPARTMENT SUBPROJECT

Introduction

A number of the problems identified in the original pilot unit involved relationships with the various clinical services departments such as pathology, radiology, and the blood bank. Therefore starting in November of 1976, Dan Hartman, one of the project consultants, met with several clinical services administrators to propose a possible interface with patient care units. The director of clinical services, Jack Mauer, who reported to the hospital director and was responsible for the twenty clinical services departments, became interested in linking up with the QWL project.

By the late spring of 1977, two distinct project activities had begun in clinical services. First, a survey feedback project was initiated in the clinical services departments to make intraservice diagnoses and promote change. Second, a task force was set up to conduct *organizational mirroring,* the exchange of information about intergroup problems between a set of six patient care units and several clinical services departments. In time, the two activities became completely independent and so will be discussed separately.

As originally conceived by Hartman and Mauer, the feedback project had several facets. First, an attitude survey would be used to ascertain initial conditions in each service. The plan was to distribute an eighty-item questionnaire to measure trust, decision making, communication, satisfaction, work group functioning, and superior-subordinate relationships. Employees within each service would fill out the questionnaire.

The plan was presented at a meeting of the clinical services department heads in March of 1977, and—although several doctors and administrators commented that such projects had been conducted before without any substantial results—the group decided to proceed with the project. It lasted for almost two years.

The Columbia research team became involved in the clinical services subproject at its inception. We were looking forward to studying a new area of the hospital, and our participation was facilitated by the fact that the project had a built-in evaluation component: We would design the main pretest questionnaire, provide the results, and then perform the follow-up, posttest data collection. The analysis plan called for a comparison of control services (those which received no feedback) and experimental services (those which used the feedback in problem-solving activities).

In May of 1977 the department heads and their representatives were briefed on the administration of the newly designed survey questionnaire. Feedback was planned for the following month, but the project fell behind. By July of 1977, Steve Meyer had replaced Dan Hartman, who had left the consulting group, and a new timetable (see Figure 10.3) was prepared for future activities. They included the selection and training of facilitators to work with the directors in providing the feedback and preparing action plans for change.

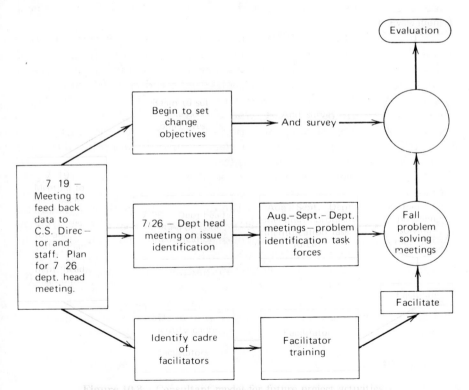

Figure 10.3. Consultant model for future project activities.

By this point the complexity of monitoring the project had increased. It appeared that the project would span about two years, involve fourteen departments, and have an evolving, ambiguous set of goals and roles. We developed facilitator log books so we would have a record of what happened in each department at each feedback meeting. It had become impossible for us to monitor all activities, and we hoped the log books would fill the gaps in our own observations.

On August 25, 1977, the department heads met to look at their data. The results had been put in chart form and included a comparison of the department mean to the total sample mean on each variable. (See Figure 10.4.) During the fall it seemed that the project was moving slowly, and that not all experimental services were involved in the same activities. Some departments met and solved problems, while others didn't meet at all. Some facilitators and directors were active, but some did nothing. We realized that we would have to make department-by-department determinations regarding whether or not feedback had been presented and used and might therefore yield positive change.

Then in January of 1978, the director of clinical services decided that facilitators should switch departments. Not all of them changed, but those who were administrators in a particular service became facilitators there so that project activities could be built into regular unit functioning. At this point the director's involvement in the project decreased to almost nothing, and activity by the facilitators either ceased or became an integral part of administrative functioning. Four departments dropped out of the project completely and refused to allow the administration of a second questionnaire.

We still, however, planned to make hypotheses about change in the departments. To do so, we combined observation results with semistructured interviews with the director, the facilitators, and departmental administrators. Lastly, we decided to add questions to the final questionnaire asking respondents to explicitly rate the use of feedback and the results that were achieved.

In all, we used four data collection methods. These included survey data collection and analysis of two waves of data, facilitator log books, semistructured interviews with department heads, and observation and documentation of meetings. Each of these will be discussed separately.

Questionnaires

In the early summer of 1977 and again in the summer of 1978, questionnaires were administered in the fourteen designated clinical serv-

Key: H = high agreement among employee responses
M = moderate agreement among employee responses
L = low agreement among employee responses

Importance of Factors Influencing Job Satisfaction

How important is:	Dept. Mean	Dept. Agree.	Means 1 2 3 4 5	Total Mean	Total Agree.
1. Friendliness of others	3.90	M		3.50	M
2. Fringe benefits	4.33	H		3.94	M
3. Respect from others	4.15	H		4.08	M
4. Chances to accomplish	4.28	M		4.21	M
5. Amount of pay	4.47	H		4.19	H
6. Hours you work	3.30	L		3.51	M
7. Way you are treated	4.33	H		4.06	M
8. Chances for getting ahead	3.69	M		3.60	M
9. Amount of security	4.23	M		4.14	M
10. Opportunity to develop yourself	4.31	M		4.32	M
11. Cooperation from co-workers	4.10	M		4.10	M

Satisfaction with Job Factors

How satisfied are you with:	Dept. Mean	Dept. Agree	Means 1 2 3 4 5	Total Mean	Total Agree.
1. Friendliness of others	4.00	M		3.75	M
2. Fringe benefits	3.62	L		3.83	M
3. Respect from others	3.80	M		3.70	M
4. Chances to accomplish	3.26	M		3.27	M
5. Amount of pay	3.18	M		3.23	M
6. Chances to do something worthwhile	3.39	M		3.67	M
7. Way you are treated	3.77	M		3.63	M
8. Chances for getting ahead	2.69	M		2.71	M
9. Job security	3.17	M		3.46	M
10. Opportunity to develop yourself	3.21	M		2.98	M
11. Hours you work	4.26	M		4.09	M
12. Cooperation from co-workers	3.77	M		3.58	M
13. Information on what's happening at Parkside	2.45	M		2.78	M
14. Training you received	3.51	L		3.37	M
15. Your department chief	4.03	M		3.51	M

Figure 10.4. Sample of Survey Feedback Given to Departments: Clinical Services Survey, Parkside Hospital (Broken lines =Dept. Mean, Solid lines =Total Mean)

201

ices departments. The first wave results constituted the major source of feedback for service diagnosis and problem solving. They also served as a baseline measure to which the second wave could be compared for pinpointing improvement in the departments.

The questionnaire was a modified version of the Michigan Organizational Assessment Questionnaire (Cammann, Fichman, Jenkins, & Kelsh, 1983). Specific modules and scales were selected based on their relevance to the setting and nature of the project, and therefore the modules differed slightly from the pilot unit questionnaire. Also, several additional items were included at the request of one of the project consultants.

The final clinical services questionnaire contained 120 items, most of which called for responses on a five-point Likert-type scale ranging from (1) "to a very little extent" or (1) "disagree" to (5) "to a very great extent" or (5) "agree." As noted above, additional items were added to the questionnaire for the second administration to tap employee perceptions of how useful the survey feedback project had been for them.

Questionnaires were handed out to employees on all shifts. They were returned via drop boxes. Participation was voluntary, and confidentiality was insured. The first questionnaire yielded 354 respondents, while the second yielded only 216. However, four departments had dropped out of the project between the first and second administrations.

Varimax factor analysis was performed on the modules of the Michigan Organizational Assessment Questionnaire to verify the instrument's intended structure and to compute scales. In addition to the resulting twenty-three scales, three questionnaire items which did not load on any factor were kept in the analysis, separately. Table 10.7 lists these items, the twenty-three scales, their reliability coefficients (Chronbach's α) and identifies which of the full array of twenty-six measures would be most likely to be affected if the project were a success.

By reviewing the facilitator log books, the interview results, and the evaluation team's observations, it was possible to predict the direction of change for each of the clinical services departments. Table 10-8 reports the predicted change, as well as the predicted source of the change. We predicted that there would be changes only in the blood bank, chemistry, library, and radiology. Changes would reflect both project and nonproject related activities.

Once the scales had been calculated, t-tests for each clinical services department, comparing its scores on all scales prior to the project (T1 = summer 1977) and after the end of all project activities (T2 = sum-

Table 10.7. Clinical Services Project Questionnaire Scales

		Coefficient α	# items	Predictions of Project Impact
1.	Importance of co-workers	.78	4	−
2.	Importance of extrinsic rewards	.71	4	−
3.	Importance of achievement	.82	4	−
4.	Satisfaction with co-workers	.93	4	+
5.	Satisfaction with extrinsic rewards	.60	2	−
6.	Satisfaction with achievement	.83	6	+
7.	If do job well, greater extrinsic rewards	.75	4	−
8.	If do a poor job, someone will get angry at you	single item		+
9.	If do job poorly, co-workers help	.63	2	+
10.	If do job well, greater sense of achievement	.80	2	−
11.	Freedom on the job	.83	5	+
12.	Variety on the job	.71	2	−
13.*	Not enough time to get work done	.78	3	+
14.	Work group listens and trusts	.89	7	+
15.	Work group is competent	.88	6	+
16.*	No matter what, others criticize you	single item		+
17.*	Conflict between groups	.89	3	+
18.	Discuss problems with other groups	.88	2	+
19.	Different groups work well with each other	single item		+
20.	Supervisor listens, encourages, sets example	.89	8	+
21.	Director listens, encourages, sets example	.90	7	+
22.	Director is informed of department activities	.82	3	+
23.	Have a say in how to do work	.91	4	+
24.	Have a say in policies	.79	5	−
25.	Hospital is improving	.81	6	+
26.	Satisfaction with working at Parkside	.85	2	+

Notes.
*reverse scaling
+ indicates that if project was a success, these scales could improve.
− project not expected to impact

mer 1978), were run. This was done to test for attitudinal and percep-
tual change in each department in the interim period. The two samples
were obviously not independent, since it was a test-retest design. This
made it more difficult to obtain significant differences. Although the
original data analysis plan called for a comparison of control services
(those which received no feedback) and experimental services (those
which used the feedback in various ways), this design became impossible to implement. The sample size of the experimental units was very
small, and services contained both those staff members who had received the feedback and those who had not. Therefore the original design was dropped, and only T1 and T2 scores for each department were
compared. The results of the test are given in Tables 10.8 and 10.9 and

Table 10.8.   Predicted and Actual Directions and Sources of Change in the
Clinical Services Departments

Predictions of Change	Source		Actual Results
Blood Bank			
Positive	Project—Talked over issues, feedback resulted in regular meetings	18	scale scores improve
	Nonproject—reorganization of department	8	scale scores decline
	Organizational mirroring project	3	scale scores significantly improved[a]
	New office arrangements		
	New telephone system		
	New administration		
Chemistry			
Positive or none	Project—In-service education program started.	3	scale scores improve
	After initial meetings had them stopped because not seen as ben-eficial.	23	scale scores decline
	Nonproject—New chairman	3	scale scores significantly decline
Library			
None or negative	Project—Meetings held but peo-ple got cynical when a lot of time was spent at meetings with little results	17	scale scores improve
		9	scale scores decline
		3	scale scores significantly decline

Table 10.8. (Continued)

Predictions of Change	Source	Actual Results	
Microbiology			
None	Project—Feedback given but no need seen for more meetings since employees saw problems as institution-wide and nothing could be done	11	scale scores improve
		15	scale scores decline
		1	scale score significantly improves
Pathology			
None	Project—Results reported but meetings ended because people thought they were a waste of time	16	scale scores improve
		10	scale scores decline no scale scores significantly changed
Radiology			
Positive change	Project—Feedback in May 1978 Nonproject—New chairman New departmental structure Four supervisors replaced	19	scale scores improve
		7	scale scores decline no scale scores significantly changed
Radiotherapy			
None	Project—No feedback	17	scale scores improve
		9	scale scores decline no scale scores significantly changed
Rehabilitation medicine			
??	No one could say—Had lost track after limited exposure	10	scale scores improve
		16	scale scores decline no scale scores significantly changed
Respiratory therapy			
none	Project—Discussions about managers who were gone by the time of the survey	10	scale scores improve
		16	scale scores decline no scale scores significantly changed

Note. a significant $p = < .05$ (1-tailed test).

205

Table 10.9. *T*-Tests for Each Department—Time 1 vs. Time 2

					Department					
Scale	Bloodbk	Chem	Library	Mibiol	Nukemed	Pathol	Radiol	Rther	Rehabm	Respira
1			.060*							
2										
3				0.53*						
4			.025	.046–			.002			
5				.008–						
6										
7										
8		.023–								
9		.054–*								
10		.000–	.067*–					.032–	.068–	
11		.008–								
12		.100–*					.01			
13										

14					
15	.094*				.001
16	.061*	.067*−			.003
17					
18	.011		.083−*		
19	.097*				
20				.001	
21				.002−	
22				.017−	
23				.044	
24	.024				
25	.005				
26					

*significant if 1-tailed test used

−becomes more negative over time

Note. Empty cells indicate no significant differences.

include the mean differences and t-test results for each department, on each scale, in T1 and T2.

The data showed that most of the change in attitudes occurred in the blood bank and the chemistry and radiology departments with some minor change in the library and the microbiology department and essentially no change in the others. This closely followed predicted results except for the chemistry department, which was predicted to improve but whose scores became more negative. At T2, blood bank employees stated greater satisfaction with working at Parkside and were more inclined to agree that their work groups were competent, worked well together, and discussed problems with other groups. Chemistry department employees, on the other hand, reported less freedom on the job, less variety on the job, less of a sense of achievement if they did well, and less support from co-workers if they were doing badly. Changes in the radiology department centered around increased satisfaction with the work group and supervisor but also decreased satisfaction with the director.

Additions were made to the second questionnaire administration to tap employee perceptions of the data feedback project. In response to the question, "Have the results of the first questionnaire survey been presented to the employees in your department?" 47.7 percent said "yes," 22.6 percent said "no," and 29.6 percent didn't know. Of those who saw the results, 23.7 percent thought they were not presented clearly, 38.6 percent thought they were presented somewhat clearly, and 37.7 percent thought they were presented very clearly.

Only 4.7 percent of the respondents indicated that results were posted, while 19.8 percent indicated that they were handed out, 52.8 percent indicated that they were presented in work group meetings, and 22.6 percent indicated that they were presented in departmental meetings. When asked how the survey results were used, 39.1 percent said not at all, 34.4 percent said to air feelings and criticisms, 15.6 percent said to help solve problems, and 10.9 percent said to set goals. Fifty-seven percent said that survey results were never discussed informally, 47.2 percent said sometimes, and 5 percent said frequently. Finally, 69.6 percent rated the survey results as not at all useful, 26.1 percent rated them somewhat useful, and 4.3 percent rated them extremely useful. Table 10.10 reports the ratings on a department-by-department basis.

The data clearly indicated that some of the departments changed, but that most did not. The radiology department and the blood bank showed the most positive changes. However, they were the sites of a reorganization, staff changes, and other nonproject events which could

Table 10.10. Responses to Questions of How Data Were Communicated and How They Were Used for Clinical Services Departments

Department Responses	Number Questionnaires Returned	Results Posted	Results Handed Out	Meetings W/Work Group	Meetings W/Dept.	Results Not Used	Used to Air Feelings	Used for Prob. Solving	Used to Set Goals
Blood bank	4	—	—	1	2	—	2	2	2
Chemistry	29	3	11	6	6	10	3	5	3
Library	26	2	6	17	4	3	15	5	1
Microbiology	16	—	—	8	3	10	6	—	1
Nuclear medicine	6	—	—	—	—	—	—	—	—
Pathology	12	—	—	2	1	3	2	—	—
Radiology	75	—	10	7	2	9	5	7	3
Radiation therapy	11	—	—	1	—	5	1	1	1
Rehabilitation	21	—	1	12	6	7	8	—	1
Respiratory therapy	6	—	3	2	—	3	2	—	2
	216								

have caused the changes in questionnaire measures. The chemistry department changed in a negative direction, and the rest did not change at all. These data were consistent with the variance in how the data were fed back. The blood bank and the radiology department had problem-solving meetings or data feedback, while other departments didn't even see the data.

Facilitator Log Books

We asked the facilitators to keep a log of project activities in each department assigned to them. We provided instructions on the purpose and use of the log at the October 1977 meeting. The log books included two forms for the facilitators to fill out for each meeting: a department activity log form and a feedback meeting rating form. The former was intended to provide a capsule summary of all the meetings in any one department. It called for a list of attendees for each meeting, a short account of the meeting's purpose, key outcomes, and comments. The latter required more in-depth information on key events, outcomes, and the nature of the feedback process. It contained a questionnaire centered on the method of feedback presentation, what the feedback was used for, and how employees reacted to it. Facilitators were asked to evaluate the supervisors, employees, and themselves regarding participation and effectiveness.

Although facilitators were given very general training in data feedback and its effective use, they were not required to employ any one style or set of activities. This, coupled with different levels of facilitator training and different levels of commitment in the various departments, indicated that the individual departments would use the data in different ways.

The feedback literature (see Bowers & Franklin, 1972; Klein, Kraut, & Wolfson, 1971; Nadler, 1976, 1977) would predict different results because of the variety of feedback processes. Thus obtaining accurate information about the feedback process in each service would enable us to predict which departments would improve and which would decline. Since detailed observation of each service by the research group was impossible, we hoped that the facilitator log books would supplement key observations in providing an assessment of the feedback design implementation.

Unfortunately, only two of the five facilitators filled out their log books; the others either lost the log book, had no departmental feedback meetings, or simply were not motivated to fill out the forms. Given the scarcity of data, the log books were used only to predict changes in specific departments.

Interviews

The semistructured interviews included questions about the activities project participants were involved in, their views of the strengths and weaknesses of the project, their initial and final attitudes toward the project, and their assessment of the project's effects. Each of these will be examined separately. The facilitators, the director of clinical services, and department administrators were interviewed. In all, ten interviews were conducted. The responses were content analyzed and yielded the results that follow.

The number of participants' project roles and activities was almost as great as the number of people interviewed. The work of facilitators ranged from distributing surveys and showing the data to department heads to helping to plan feedback meetings, to facilitating meetings led by department heads, to running feedback meetings themselves. Some facilitators became closely involved with departments, while others could not get past department heads who refused to permit feedback meetings.

In all, four departments dropped out of the project completely by refusing to allow administration of the second questionnaire; two got no feedback at all (see Table 10.8), six got feedback but spent little or no time working with it; and two spent a great deal of time discussing the feedback. Of the two which made a considerable effort to use the data for discussion and problem solving, only one found the activity worth the effort.

All interviewees evaluated the strengths and weaknesses of the project. Those which were mentioned by at least three of the ten interviewed are listed below:

Major Strengths

Gave managers a sense of the type and magnitude of department problems

Provided an outlet for employees—their voice was heard

Gave positive reinforcement to departments that did well

Provided for the personal and professional growth of facilitators and managers

Brought the clinical services division together by giving facilitators a look at their counterparts in other departments and a better knowledge of their own department vis-a-vis others

Major Weaknesses

Period of tumultuousness for departments, so not a good time for the project

Director of clinical services was new and did not have firm administrative control

Project not marketed well—not seen as a high priority activity

Project not "owned" by participants; many felt pressure to become involved

Not enough active leadership

Goals unclear

No action plans—no timetables for goals

Inexperienced facilitators—not comfortable with role

Not enough training of department heads for data feedback

Project presented with too much jargon—not understood by everyone

Department heads not prepared for the time and energy commitment required

Results fed back too slowly

Items in questionnaire repeated, too general, and not in Spanish

Issues brought up but not dealt with

All those interviewed were asked about their attitudes toward the project both when they initially heard about it and a year later, in June 1978. Most of the interviewees were "cautiously optimistic" at first although two were quite overtly negative. Most believed that the project might work but had many reservations stemming primarily from their past experiences. Specifically, reservations derived from the knowledge that many previous surveys had not produced results, that the nature of the institution did not foster change, that union-management relations were poor, and that previous external consultants at the hospital had a poor achievement record. Great changes were not anticipated.

A year later, attitudes were more negative. The results were not those for which the interviewees had hoped. Most felt that some good had come out of the project, particularly the personal growth experienced by many. Nevertheless, their expectations were unfulfilled, and thus they felt that much time had been wasted. It was generally agreed that some good ideas had emerged from the project, but that hospital and departmental conditions coupled with poor implementation had aborted their implementation.

The effects perceived by the interviewees mirrored their attitudes toward the project rather well. Those individuals whose departments had done nothing saw no effects. Others felt the project had achieved a positive result by encouraging people to talk and vent feelings but noted that these were not always dealt with. These interviewees said that workers got to know managers better, and facilitators came to know individuals in their departments. However, they stated, little if any problem-solving and goal-setting activity took place—employees were brought together simply to talk.

To summarize, there were some effects in a few departments, particularly more open communication and better interpersonal relations: "but in the institution as a whole—negligible effects," to quote an interviewee. As one individual concluded, the effort will "go down with hundreds of other projects where the hospital has thrown out thousands of dollars for minimal effects."

Observation

As in much of the rest of the project, a primary data collection method was structured naturalistic observation. Meetings within the clinical services administration and those between the administration and individual departments were documented by the evaluation team in a standardized format. The identity of the observers and the date, time, and setting of the observations were noted. Key events at meetings, detailed observations, and observer interpretations and feelings were recorded separately. In addition to this documentation, handouts and minutes of past meetings kept by hospital personnel were gathered so that the history of the project would be more accurate. All of these sources were used in writing this narrative.

Discussion

It is clear that many of the objectives stated at the beginning of the clinical services subproject were not met. But most of those interviewed—persons who were involved in the planning and implementation of the project—felt that many positive results were achieved.

The objectives of the project called for (1) administering a questionnaire, (2) providing data feedback to all fourteen clinical services involved in the project, (3) identifying problem areas in the services, (4) conducting problem-solving meetings to address those issues, (5) training facilitators to assist in the above process, and (6) resurveying the services to determine (a) if positive changes had taken place in such areas as satisfaction with co-workers, achievement, work group competence, work group support, supervisors, directors, and the hospital and (b) if change toward a feeling of greater participation in and control over the work environment had occurred.

Clearly, all of these objectives were not met. Four of the services dropped out of the project before feedback was given. Six of the remaining ten were not expected to change because either feedback was not given or was seen as useless since it raised issues that could not be dealt with. Survey results indicated that, indeed, these six services showed no improvement. The remaining four departments did show change. The chemistry department showed negative change for reasons which could not be determined by the evaluation team. The library showed negative change, partially due to union-management difficulties. However, the radiology department and the blood bank did improve. Yet this improvement was due not only to their involvement in this project but also to the organizational mirroring subproject, organizational restructuring, and changes in key, high-ranking personnel. Therefore we cannot credit the clinical services subproject alone.

Regarding the original objectives, it can be seen that: (1) not all services got feedback, (2) still fewer identified problem areas to work on, and (3) even less (two) actually worked on them. Finally, only one department reported positive changes. In this department, the facilitator became the administrator for the department and incorporated the meetings into ongoing departmental activity.

Although the original objectives were not met and survey results and interviews showed little improvement in services, some positive results were obtained. Even where employees did not receive feedback, service directors did and thereby became more aware of their staff's attitudes. Employees, views and feelings received a hearing. Facilitators learned a great deal personally and professionally and assisted in communication between the various services.

Why wasn't more achieved? The participants summed up the major weaknesses of the project fairly well. At the project's start, great enthusiasm was exhibited by the director of clinical services and the original consultant team. This enthusiasm and commitment was perceived by the heads of services as pressure to join what was supposedly a volunteer project. Thus from the very beginning the project was not owned by its participants. In addition, no one was fully prepared for the time commitment that the meetings required.

As time progressed, it became clear that both service heads and facilitators were unclear about their roles in the feedback process or were insufficiently skilled to carry out those roles. As the director of clinical services became less involved in the project and abdicated leadership, the status of the project declined to a low priority activity. He saw his purpose to be getting the project off the ground and believed that the facilitators should then take over. But the facilitators, for various reasons, did not fulfill his expectations. The facilitators felt that goal time-tables and support from top management were needed to achieve the goals. The enormous time and commitment required to influence department heads was not forthcoming. Many facilitators didn't have the necessary skills, their services were not wanted, they received no external rewards for their work, and the seemingly minimal results of the project were discouraging. Although Steve Meyer tried to spur the facilitators on, there were too many forces encouraging their noninvolvement.

The failure of the facilitators was apparent after the January reshuffling of their responsibilities. Only one of them had achieved success. He was among the more skilled of the facilitators and worked in his own department—the blood bank—where he had authority. The success of his work made a difference in his job with regard to his relationships to his staff, and thus he had a sense of ownership. Therefore he was motivated to set the goals, objectives, and timetables with the help of the department staff—marketing and leadership from the director of clinical services were not needed.

THE ORGANIZATION MIRRORING SUBPROJECT

In Chapter 8 we describe a subproject which involved the Parkside blood bank, the radiology department, and several nursing units throughout the hospital. This "Organization Mirroring" subproject set up a two-way communications process that was intended to improve the coordination between the clinical services and the department of nursing and to lessen the antagonism between them.

Methods

At the beginning of the project, the question of who would be responsible for gathering data on the two mirroring sites was discussed with the QWL steering committee. Since this was planned as an action research project in which data collection and analysis would be an intergral part of the total intervention, the Columbia research team took a passive observational role. In March of 1978, after considerable discussion, the responsibility for developing quantitative measures of the outcomes of the two site-level projects was given jointly to the director of nursing, the director of clinical services, the director of research for the nursing department, and the consultant, Bill Evans. In the end, none of those who was given responsibility produced a viable measurement strategy. As a result, the two pilot site projects were left to determine their own means of evaluation. The data that were generated by the project site teams proved to be essentially worthless from an assessment perspective.

Given the absence of "hard" data, observation became the main source of assessment data for the mirroring project. The two pilot projects were monitored by Columbia research team observers who attended almost all of the groups' meetings. Observational data were recorded in a standardized format using the methods of structured naturalistic observation (Nadler, Perkins, & Hanlon, 1983). The data recording categories included key events, detailed observations, interpretive material, and the observer's affective reactions to the observed events. In addition, an assessment of group process was done using a formal process evaluation form. Minutes taken by group members were also included. Open-ended, unstructured interviews with participants of the two pilot projects were carried out at random intervals during the course of the projects. Finally, interviews were carried out after the termination of the two pilot projects. In these interviews, the Columbia research team member provided his or her assessment of project results, and the interviewee was invited to comment on the extent to which these assessment perceptions were correct.

Results

The major outcomes of the blood bank and radiology department projects are presented in narrative form in Chapter 8. Both projects were successful in proposing and implementing useful changes in work procedures. The projects demonstrated that interdepartmental, multilevel working groups could be created to deal with a common set of problems. At times, both groups functioned very well; problems were identified and procedural changes were suggested and implemented. In the radiology department, a new procedure for delivering x-rays to different parts of the hospital was implemented successfully. The groups did communicate to one another about problems in their divisions, so that even if all problems were not solved, a better understanding of the other division was achieved for committee members. The groups demonstrated the potential that the QWL project could have had at Parkside.

But despite their achievements, neither group survived beyond the end of the pilot phase. As we note in Chapter 8, responsibility for the demise of these projects rests with the senior management of the nursing and clinical services departments. Without support from above, continuation of the projects beyond the tenure of the consultants was not possible.

Finally, part of the blame must lie with the consultants. Once the two pilot projects were up and moving, the consultants spent less and less time with them. By the time the project members had completed their initial work, the consultants had left the hospital. The consultants had not, however, put any structures in place to assure project continuity. They did not meet with the steering committee to discuss its future role, nor did they inform the pilot groups how to carry on once their initial work was done. Thus the project demonstrates once again an intervention that led to individual growth, new skill development and improved hospital procedures. It did not, however, institutionalize the change or the change process, and mirroring activity ceased.

CHAPTER ELEVEN

Learning from Parkside
Quality of Work Life Reform in Health Care Settings

The Parkside Quality of Work Life Project ended formally in 1978. Over the course of the following year and into 1980, the research team continued to visit the hospital to collect data for the final report on the project, which was submitted to the funding agency in the spring of 1980. Although less than two years had elapsed since the last steering committee meeting, we found that the project existed only in the memories of the participants—those who could be found, we should say. Parkside continued to experience a high turnover of staff, and several of the major figures in the QWL project had left the hospital.

But there is more to the story. In early 1982, Harvey Hertz, who had been elevated to the title of President of Parkside Medical Center, contacted one of the authors and asked for help in planning an effort to improve patient care in the hospital. The author returned to the hospital and with colleagues, developed some strategic planning options for the hospital. The course of this consultation went beyond the issues addressed by the Parkside project. But the opportunity to return to Parkside and to take a second look allowed us to explore some of the deeper questions about the suitability of the QWL model in large medical care settings. It also allowed us to investigate why the project received so little support despite the tremendous show of enthusiasm on the part of management (and the unions) at the beginning and the manifest need to improve the quality of work life in the hospital.

In this chapter, we approach the ultimate failure of the Parkside project in three ways. First, we analyze Parkside using an evaluative model derived from a comparative research project that was carried out by two of the authors of this book. Our emphasis here is on identi-

219

fying the specific factors that account for the limited and short-lived effects of the Parkside project. Second, we present some of the findings of the diagnostic activities from the 1982 venture. Here the emphasis is on the problematic relationship between the QWL project and its democratic, cooperative philosophy and the turbulent organizational climate within the hospital at the time of the project. These observations form the basis for our third concern in this chapter, the ultimate question of whether the quality of work life model can be made appropriate to complex health care settings.

A PREDICTIVE MODEL OF QUALITY OF WORK LIFE PROJECT SUCCESS

In a comparative study of sixteen joint labor-management quality of work life projects, Nadler, Hanlon, and Lawler (1980) specified five factors—essentially corollaries of Walton and McKersie's (1965) integrative barganining model—that determine project outcomes. The five factors are summarized in Figure 11.1.

The first factor is "ownership" of the project by union and management, or the felt commitment to the concept and goals of a QWL project. Clarity of goals is the second factor; the rewards for involvement are greater when the goals are clear, tangible, and agreed upon by both sides. The effectiveness of the external consultant is the third factor. The consultant or consultant team is particularly important in the early stages of a QWL project, during the period when trust between union and management and the informal channels of communication remain undeveloped. The consultant plays a key transitional role in facilitating communication and building trust. The fourth factor is the labor-management committee and its effectiveness as a vehicle for integrative bargaining. The composition of the committee is especially important; it must include representatives with sufficient authority to institutionalize work reforms that come out of QWL project activity. Finally, the organizational context is crucial. This includes two major elements: the prevailing labor relations climate and the organization's financial status. These five factors were derived empirically and were related significantly to evaluations of overall project success across the sample of sixteen QWL projects (see Nadler, Hanlon, & Lawler, 1980).

Clearly, these factors fit the Parkside case as well. Ownership was a crucial issue. None of the parties was required to provide tangible support or significant funds for the project. It was a free good. The representative from the National Quality of Work Center who introduced the project to the union and to the hospital minimized its costs and

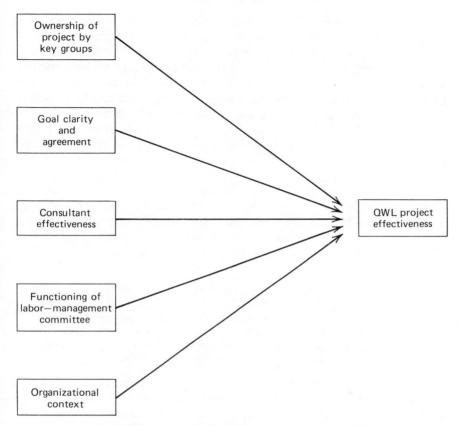

Figure 11.1 Determinants of QWL project outcomes.

risks by portraying the project only in the most vague, general, and positive terms. The result of what was basically a conflict avoidance strategy was the creation of a situation in which participants did not have a sense of what would be asked of them and what could be expected in return. A typical perception was:

> I was invited to a meeting with a representative from an organization in Washington, D.C. . . . I listened and I heard somebody had some money they wanted to spend, and they were going to study a quality of work situation in a hospital, and the one thing I was sure of was that there was a need to improve the quality of work in the hospital.

During this vague, ambiguous period, several critical decisions were made that shaped the course of the project. Without much in the way of critical consideration, the decision was made to make a patient care unit the focal point of the project. This had one strategic advantage: All disciplines and unions were represented on patient care units. But in retrospect, the decision created extremely difficult problems for the consultants and the project steering committee. A patient care unit is highly dependent upon several hospital functions, and this fact made it difficult to carry out substantive work reforms. Also, a unit-based project does not involve major figures in the hospital—both union and management. The project started off small, weak, and constrained by the dependence of the unit upon the larger support system of the hospital.

Thus the start-up phase created a legacy of ambiguity, poor site selection, and a lack of goal clarity and commitment to the project. And as we describe in Chapter 4, the structure and function of the union-management steering committee was never made clear. This was in turn a major reason for its ineffectiveness. As one committee member noted:

> For a long time, the people on the steering committee didn't know what they were or what they were there for, or what they were supposed to do. At some of the meetings I almost felt like I was an experimental animal in a cage being watched, because obviously they were putting us in this position and purposely letting us find our way, and we didn't know how to find our way too well, so we were inefficient and wasted a lot of time.

Consultant incompetence was a major problem in the case of the first consulting team. It is important to note that consultant team members enjoyed considerable reputations as traditional management consultants. But this was not a traditional consulting situation, and the team appeared as lost as everyone else in the crucial early days of the project. The second consulting team was, by consensus, competent, well-liked, and provided a much needed source of energy. But they arrived near the midpoint of the project's life span, when a significant share of the external funds had been depleted and strategic decisions about the focus of the project had already been made. The consultants were forced to undo much of the old while trying to build up a project that made sense. In the end, they were overwhelmed by the project.

Finally it is essential to consider the last factor in the predictive model described above—the organizational context. The troubled state of union-management relations at the time of the project should be clear from the narrative. Here our focus is on how the financial problems that plagued the hospital at the time of the project and the management reforms that were carried out to ameliorate these problems affected the project's course. Data are from the 1982 follow-up research. The central figure is Harvey Hertz, the president of the hospital.

By early 1982, Hertz had completed the extensive reformation of the financial and management systems of the hospital that was started during the initial phase of the QWL project. He felt that he had carried out this difficult task successfully—a point of view shared by knowledgeable observers both within and outside of the hospital. He commented to a member of the original research team that:

> If we look at the goals we had in 1975, we have made progress in most of the key areas. We have built financial stability, we are doing better planning, and we are working out the physical redesign of the hospital.

He noted, however, that:

> My one biggest frustration is that we have not made progress on improving employee attitudes and patient care. Many of our employees feel that this is not a good place to work. Many of our patients feel that they are not treated well.

Soon after, a three-person consulting team which included one of the original researchers was assembled to carry out a comprehensive diagnostic survey of the hospital. The objective was to identify means of improving patient care and staff attitudes. The consulting team worked closely with an internal team headed by Parkside's recently appointed vice-president of human resources.

The diagnosis was carried out within the framework of a specific organizational assessment model (see Nadler & Tushman, 1982 for a description). The major findings were as follows:

> In 1975, Hertz arrived to find the hospital fundamentally out of control. The institution was faced with mounting operating deficits, and the existing management had little awareness of how funds were being spent or how to control costs. Moreover, the physician-dominated culture was hostile to the idea of management accountability.

> Soon after, Hertz collected data and developed his basic strategy, which involved the establishment of management control by building information systems, developing a financial planning system, and setting a specific goal to operate the hospital on a break-even basis. The basic work of patient care, teaching, and research would be carried out within the framework of this fiscal management goal.

The hospital's organization was changed into a matrix form which strengthened the roles of functional department heads in nursing, clinical services, and support services. A new top management group, labelled the Senior Management Group or SMG, was created as a focal point for management decision making. A project management system was begun to track different initiatives and activities.

An informal organization was also developed which supported the formal organizational changes. A "professional management" perspective rather than a medical perspective pervaded the climate of senior management. A more confrontational and adversarial climate was created to encourage more critical review of actions. These initiatives, combined with existing conflicts between disciplines and demographic differences (race, ethnicity, sex), intensified intergroup conflict within the hospital. This was acceptable to Hertz, since the focus of the strategy was control of the activities within each department of the hospital, not cooperation between departments. Managers were rewarded for the performance of their own units in financial terms rather on their record in promoting linkages to other units.

Hertz brought in several new senior managers who shared his perspective and values. Managers who did not accept the new strategy were encouraged to leave.

In short, Hertz was involved in a major effort to establish a professional management culture in a setting that was dominated by health care professionals with little management training or background and a profound lack of interest in financial or organizational accountability. His goal was to bring a large measure of rationalization to the "doctor's workshop." These changes had the intended effect upon the financial performance of the hospital. They did not, however, provide a setting that was conducive to attempts to improve patient care such as the Parkside Quality of Work Life Project.

The QWL project was intended to decentralize decision making while Hertz was attempting to centralize control. The project focused on patient care while Hertz refocused the organization in the direction of better financial performance. The project attempted to foster collaboration across departmental boundaries; Hertz sought to strengthen boundaries in order to define manageable units and areas of responsibility. The project strove for union-management cooperation while Hertz's financial strategy demanded an "arms-length" and often highly adversarial stance toward the unions. In sum, Hertz was creating an environment that was hostile to the aims of the project.

It is important to note that Hertz's strategy is not an unusual one for large, not-for-profit hospitals that are struggling to maintain their share of the medical care market place in an era of escalating costs, external regulations, and increased competition from other forms of health care organizations—notably, proprietary hospital chains. Indeed, the pressure to rationalize, to impose the stamp of management on the loosely coupled operations of large medical centers is one of the most significant trends in the health care industry today. If Hertz was exceptional it was only because his efforts were largely successful. But by the time of our return to the hospital in 1982, the "downside" of this strategy was apparent in the continuing crisis of patient care, poor morale among staff, and (significantly) Hertz's new receptivity to the idea of a quality of work life project.

Given its marginal status within the chief administrator's strategic plan, the Parkside QWL Project *was never given the resources that were essential to address the major structural causes of the hospital's problems.* The diagnosis carried out in 1982 identified structural factors as perhaps the most critical problem regarding patient care. The hospital had been structured in a way that did not support patient care. The control strategy that Hertz developed required a structure in which individual functions and responsibilities could be identified and measured. A structure that supported patient care would be oriented toward sets of patients with similar needs and would encourage collaboration among the different groups (managers, physicians, nurses, technicians, and support staff) that provided care to this set of patients. In brief, the hospital had been organized around the work of control rather than the work of caring for patients.

In 1982, the consultants saw this issue as critical. They felt that any major reorganization in the interest of improved patient care would require a significant restructuring of the organizational units of the hospital.

Thus if one were to examine the different problems identified throughout the course of the QWL project and in the years after its termination, one would find that few problems originated within a single hospital unit—the initial focal point of the Parkside project. The problems of the unit were a result of a larger system facing a crisis of survival and going through a painful process of adaption and change. The existing informal organization, the adversarial relationships among professional groups, the lack of rewards for patient care, and the growing climate of contention were all manifestations of the changes that were occurring throughout the entire system. The basic fallacy of the project viewed from this context was that a set of activities within a small unit embedded within a larger system could succeed in addressing some of the core problems of that larger system.

As we noted earlier, successful innovations such as many of the reforms on Barnard 5 and the outcomes of the organizational mirroring projects in the radiology and blood bank departments received no external support and eventually withered away. These sites became "innovation ghettos," to use Toch and Grant's (1982) term—places that were sheltered enough to enable employees to come up with useful, often creative solutions to immediate work place problems but too isolated from centers of authority to lead to diffusion or institutionalization.

The course of the Parkside project suggests some general observations about the future of QWL programs in health care settings. First, attempts to improve organizational effectiveness that stress rationalization and greater management control create an infertile setting for quality of work life interventions. There is a fundamental contradiction between the top-down strong management approach and the bottom-up QWL approach; these paradigms cannot coexist successfully. Second, the Parkside project illustrates the importance of timing. In a retrospective comment, the director of the hospital told us, "The project was several years too early." His comment, which is borne out by our experience in other health care settings, implies that collaborative efforts to improve patient care and quality of work life are feasible only when more basic organizational objectives (such as financial stability, solving the problem of conflicting priorities, and the development of a strategic planning capability), have been met. Humanizing a bureaucracy through QWL is difficult; humanizing an incomplete bureaucracy is much more so.

A final observation on the role of unions: Our beliefs about the difficulties of the QWL approach during periods of fiscal stress apply also to union-management collaboration. In the case of Parkside, union involvement was so tenuous that it is difficult to specify what could have been different if conditions had been more benign. But there is enough accumulated evidence from other settings to show how and under what conditions unions can benefit from and contribute to quality of work life problems. A few "if onlys" should suffice here. A collaborative relationship between unions and management is possible only when the job security of the union membership is considered, if not assured. Clearly, this was not the case at Parkside. As we describe in the narrative, the threat of layoffs made it extremely difficult for the principal union representative to play a role in the joint union-management steering committee and it explained, at least in part, his erratic behavior during the course of the project. Finally, QWL programs must frame the abstract goal of improving quality of work life in terms of objectives that matter to the union. The hospital workers were very committed to the idea of career upgrading, for example, and a training program based on the specific objective of opening up new career possibilities would have been an excellent way of building commitment to the quality of work life project.

APPENDIX

Sample Documentation

CONSULTANT ORGANIZATIONAL DEVELOPMENT PLAN—PARKSIDE HOSPITAL: NATIONAL QUALITY OF WORK LIFE PROJECT

This proposal focuses on the implementation and follow through of a long lasting organizational improvement strategy initially for Barnard 5 and eventually for the total Parkside system. The emphasis is on gaining acceptance, ownership, and commitment throughout the unit and hospital for continued organizational improvement efforts.

Objective

The overall objective of the project is to help hospital personnel improve the health care delivery process and the quality of working life by affecting the organizational functioning of Barnard 5 and the Parkside system.

Specifically, we expect to:

1. Develop health care improvement teams on Barnard 5 to plan and implement organizational improvement strategies.
2. Train individual team members to use applied behavioral science skills and techniques throughout the Parkside system. The focus will be on increasing skills in problem solving, communications, supervision, group decision making and conflict resolution.
3. Create an ongoing cross-ward and cross-department consultation process in which members of the ward team and steering committee can be used by others to provide additional help

229

in planning and implementing organizational improvement efforts.

4.   Further develop the steering committee as facilitators of change in the total Parkside system—emphasizing the maintenance and diffusion of the change process.

Model for Change

Our organizational development model follows the sequence below:

	Scouting	
	Entry	
Feedback loop	Diagnosis	
	Planning	
		Feedback loop
	Action	
	Evaluation	
	Termination	

Scouting

During this phase we will be in the hospital talking with people at all levels to collect the following types of information:

1.   Major resources
2.   Major limitations
3.   Important social and cultural norms and values
4.   Major subsystems within the overall system
5.   Close relationships among major subsystems
6.   Attitudes toward change, authority, outsiders
7.   Relationship between client system and other systems in its environment . . . competitors, neighbors, regulating agencies
8.   Motivation of the client system to improve itself

Entry

During this phase the consultants will be working with the client system in developing a contract. The contract will define how the succeeding stages of the planned change process will be carried out. The emphasis is on a continuing process of sharing the expectations of the consultants and the client systems and agreeing on the contributions to be made by both parties.

Diagnosis

Because of previous diagnostic efforts by the University of Michigan and Wheaton Associates, this part of our consultation will be kept to a minimum. However, some additional diagnosis will be needed and will take place through interviews in the ward with small homogeneous groups. The reason for this approach is to encourage the participation of all members of the unit.

Planning

Planning will take place at all stages during the project. The creation of plans for change will be a cooperative activity between the client and the consultant group. The first planning step is to define the specific behavioral objectives to be achieved by the change. Once these have been established, alternative strategies or solutions can be generated.

Action

In the action phase, change strategies developed in the planning stage are implemented. The model is a dynamic model, and therefore action will occur throughout the consultation.

Evaluation

Evaluation is based on the specific objectives defined in the planning stage. We will be working closely with Columbia University in developing means to measure the extent to which objectives are accomplished.

Termination

The consultants' ultimate objective is to bring about some permanent improvement in the client system's ability to function by itself. Our diffusion strategy is intended to leave the client system with the capability of maintaining the organization improvement changes.

Basic Philosophy of Intervention

Our basic philosophy of intervention involves an action research approach. After a diagnosis is conducted, change goals and a strategy will be mutually established by the consultants and client. Expected problem areas might include interpersonal skills, group and intergroup issues, job design, systems issues and structural issues. The implementation of the change strategies will heavily involve members of the client system to facilitate their ability to implement future changes on their own.

PATIENT UNIT QUESTIONNAIRE

To Parkside Employees:

This questionnaire is being used to find out what it's like to work at Parkside Hospital and in your unit. The results of this survey will be used by researchers at Columbia University who are looking at the impact of the Quality of Work Life Project, a joint labor-management program here at Parkside.

Some of you may have filled out this questionnaire last year. We are administering the questionnaire again to help us find out how things may have changed here at Parkside since that time.

Some of the questions are factual, asking you to agree or disagree with a description of things here at Parkside. Other questions ask for your views and opinions. This is *not* a test, and there are no right or wrong answers. For the survey to be useful, it is important that you answer each question frankly and honestly.

You will notice that some of the same questions are asked several ways. This is not meant to trick you. We do this to test how well our different questions measure the same ideas. All we ask of you is that you answer each question as carefully and frankly as possible.

Your answers are *completely confidential*. No one in this organization will ever have access to information from the survey about any individual or about his or her answers. All questionnaires will be taken to Columbia University for analysis and safekeeping. Only statistical summaries for groups or sets of people will be reported.

Thank you in advance for your cooperation. We hope that you will find this questionnaire interesting and thought-provoking.

The Columbia Research Team

Introduction

First, we would like to ask you a few questions about your background to help us to compare different groups of people here at Parkside.

1.   What is your job title here at Parkside?
   - (1)   Nurse (RN)
   - (2)   Nurse (LPN)   1:15
   - (3)   Nurses aide/assistant

(4)   Unit clerk

(5)   Housekeeping

(6)   Physician (faculty, attending)

(7)   Physician (resident, intern)

(8)   Other (specify) _____

2.   In what year did you first come to work at Parkside?
     19___

3.   Do you work on (*name of unit*) most of the time?
     (1)   Yes ____
     (2)   No ____   If no: Which unit? _____

4.   What shift do you work most of the time?
     (1)   7:00 A.M.–3:00 P.M. (day)
     (2)   3:00 P.M.–11:00 P.M. (evening)
     (3)   11:00 P.M.–7:00 A.M. (night)

In this question, pleae indicate HOW
SATISFIED you are with each of the
following aspects of your job.

HOW SATISFIED ARE YOU WITH . . .

	Very Dissatisfied	Dissatisfied	Slightly Dissatisfied	Neither Satisfied nor Dissatisfied	Slightly Satisfied	Satisfied	Very Satisfied
a. ... the fringe benefits you receive? ..	[1]	[2]	[3]	[4]	[5]	[6]	[7]
b. ... the friendliness of the people you work with?	[1]	[2]	[3]	[4]	[5]	[6]	[7]
c. ... the respect you receive from the people you work with?	[1]	[2]	[3]	[4]	[5]	[6]	[7]
d. ... the chances you have to accomplish something worthwhile?	[1]	[2]	[3]	[4]	[5]	[6]	[7]
e. ... the amount of pay you get?	[1]	[2]	[3]	[4]	[5]	[6]	[7]
f. ... the chances you have to do something that makes you feel good about yourself as a person?	[1]	[2]	[3]	[4]	[5]	[6]	[7]
g. ... the way you are treated by the people you work with?	[1]	[2]	[3]	[4]	[5]	[6]	[7]
h. ... your chances for getting ahead in this organization?	[1]	[2]	[3]	[4]	[5]	[6]	[7]
i. ... the amount of job security you have?	[1]	[2]	[3]	[4]	[5]	[6]	[7]
j. ... the opportunity to develop your skills and abilities?	[1]	[2]	[3]	[4]	[5]	[6]	[7]

k. . . . the hours you have to work? . . . . . [1] [2] [3] [4] [5] [6] [7]

l. . . . the cooperation you get from   [1] [2] [3] [4] [5] [6] [7]
    coworkers? . . . .

Here are some things that could happen to you when you do your job especially well. HOW LIKELY IS IT THAT EACH OF THESE THINGS WOULD HAPPEN IF YOU DID YOUR JOB ESPECIALLY WELL?

Not At All Likely   *Somewhat Likely*   *Quite Likely*   *Extremely Likely*

a. You will get an award or pay increase.   [1] [2] [3] [4] [5] [6] [7]

b. You will feel better about yourself as a person. . . . .   [1] [2] [3] [4] [5] [6] [7]

c. You will have an opportunity to develop your skills and abilities. . . . .   [1] [2] [3] [4] [5] [6] [7]

d. You will have better job security. . . . .   [1] [2] [3] [4] [5] [6] [7]

e. You will be promoted or get a better job. . . . .   [1] [2] [3] [4] [5] [6] [7]

f. You will get a feeling that you've accomplished something worthwhile. . . .   [1] [2] [3] [4] [5] [6] [7]

Here are somethings that could happen to you if you did your job especially poorly. HOW LIKELY IS IT THAT EACH OF THESE THINGS WOULD HAPPEN IF YOU DID A POOR JOB?

Not At All Likely   *Somewhat Likely*   *Quite Likely*   *Extremely Likely*

a. Someone will get angry at you. . . . . . .   [1] [2] [3] [4] [5] [6] [7]

b. Nobody will notice. . . . .   [1] [2] [3] [4] [5] [6] [7]

c. Coworkers will help you to do a better job. . . . .   [1] [2] [3] [4] [5] [6] [7]

d. You will feel bad. . . . .   [1] [2] [3] [4] [5] [6] [7]

e. Your co-workers will have to do more work. . . . .   [1] [2] [3] [4] [5] [6] [7]

This section asks about how decisions are made here at Parkside. It is also concerned with how much influence you have over decisions that are made here.

As in other parts, read the directions in the boxes and answer the questions by checking the numbers.

Here is a list of decisions which get made at work. For each of the following decisions, PLEASE INDICATE HOW MUCH SAY YOU ACTUALLY HAVE IN MAKING THESE DECISIONS.

HOW MUCH SAY DO YOU ACTUALLY HAVE IN . . .

	No Say At All	Some Say	A Good Deal of Say	A Very Great Deal of Say

a. . . . changing how you do your work? . [1] [2] [3] [4] [5] [6] [7]

b. . . . how work will be divided up among people? [1] [2] [3] [4] [5] [6] [7]

c. . . . promoting people? [1] [2] [3] [4] [5] [6] [7]

d. . . . how to handle problems you face in your work? [1] [2] [3] [4] [5] [6] [7]

e. . . . what you do day to day? [1] [2] [3] [4] [5] [6] [7]

f. . . . when people take time off? [1] [2] [3] [4] [5] [6] [7]

g. . . . what to do if you don't get what you need to do your work? [1] [2] [3] [4] [5] [6] [7]

h. . . . how you do your own work? [1] [2] [3] [4] [5] [6] [7]

i. . . . firing people? [1] [2] [3] [4] [5] [6] [7]

j. . . . what to do if someone you depend on doesn't do his or her work? [1] [2] [3] [4] [5] [6] [7]

How much do you agree or disagree with the following general statements?

Strongly Disagree / Disagree / Slightly Disagree / Neither Agree nor Disagree / Slightly Agree / Agree / Strongly Agree

a. I can modify decisions made by other people. [1] [2] [3] [4] [5] [6] [7]

b. I seldom have decisions forced on me. [1] [2] [3] [4] [5] [6] [7]

c. I have a lot of say over how decisions are made. [1] [2] [3] [4] [5] [6] [7]

SAMPLE OBSERVATION

Setting: Barnard 5   M. Hanlon
Event: Staff conference   May 12, 1977
                                                3:30–4:10 PM

Meeting to Discuss Nursing Standards

Key Events

The meeting was the second of two meetings devoted to staff opinions
about setting uniform standards for nursing care practice on the floor.
Uniform standards are a new direction for the department of nursing.

Detailed Observations

Present: Gould, Harris, Thomas, Edwards, Schuler, Angelo, Rosen,
Bradley (In-Service Nursing Trainer), Clark, Anthony, Harris, and
two observers from the Columbia research team.

Bradley started the meeting by mentioning that it would be a
follow-up to last's week meeting in which nursing staff were given the
opportunity to discuss the merits and limitations of setting nursing
care standards. She turned the floor over to Edwards who said a few
words about the importance of nursing standards.

Bruce Gould gave a little talk about what nursing standards meant
from his perspective. They would provide criteria for judging how well
the unit is working. Each nurse would now have a definite idea of what
would be expected of him or her. Gould also said that there is a need for
written procedures for new nurses coming onto the unit. Several people agreed with Gould's points. Some added supportive comments.

Harris spoke up. "The orientation for new residents is working out
great. Things are better here now (with the doctors). Providing new
nurses with the same kind of orientation would also be helpful."

Gould suggested that setting nursing standards should be carried
out within the context of the quality of work life project.

Susan Clark gave a long talk about some of the problems involved in
setting nursing standards. She argued that standards tend to become
inflexible with time and lose their usefulness. Rosen, Gould, and
Harris all expressed agreement by saying that standards or guidelines
should be kept flexible.

This led to a long discussion of the definition of "modified primary
care nursing." Harris defined the concept as total patient care—from
admission to discharge. It would always include a comprehensive pa-

tient care plan. She supported the idea of primary care nursing, saying that it would take a good deal of work load off the shoulders of the senior clinical nurse. Staff would have more decision-making responsibility in patient care matters.

Although the implementation of standards would affect all staff, the emphasis was on the RNs. Several people spoke about the need to provide a formal orientation to new nurses on the unit. The residents' orientation was referred to several times as a useful model that could be used for nurses as well. Several people remarked how successful the orientation was. Schuler noted: "It's a real improvement. We don't look and say, 'Oh no. It's the first of the month again—here they come.' It's more even now."

Schuler summed up the consensus of the meeting. Nursing standards are much needed and would be welcomed by staff. But the new standards should not go the usual route of most new projects at Parkside—initiated with much fanfare and then forgotten.

The meeting broke up after Schuler spoke. No date was set for the next staff conference.

Interpretations

It was a good meeting. Several people spoke, and most were clearly interested in the subject of the meeting. People were very supportive of one another, and involved.

The residents' orientation has become very important in the minds of the staff as an example of what can be done through their own efforts. They seem very proud of the fact that the doctors are taking the orientation seriously.

It was unclear to me where the emphasis on nursing standards was coming from and how these new standards would affect work life on the unit. One major concern throughout the meeting was how these standards would affect the nurse's professional standing. Clark's negative opinions about inflexible standards seemed to carry the theme that rigidly applied standards would reduce the nurse's role to being a technician. Harris, on the other hand, defended the concept of standard setting. She seemed to be saying that objective standards would provide useful tools that would enable the nurse to set and carry out comprehensive patient care plans.

Edwards was officially in charge of the meeting but said very little. He had no influence on the course of the discussion. Bradley's comments didn't carry much weight either, even though she was cast in the role of the outside expert. But the meeting had enough life to it that formal leadership didn't seem to matter.

It's worth noting that even though there were three nursing assistants at the meeting, the discussion was directed totally to the RNs.
The three NAs said almost nothing and were ignored. I was surprised
that Gould did not try to draw them in as he usually does.

Feelings

I felt very good about the meeting and about the participants. It was
fun for me—and interesting.

References

Aiken, L. H. "Nurses." In D. Mechanic (ed.), *Handbook of Health, Health Care, and the Health Professions,* pp. 407–431. New York: The Free Press, 1983.

Alderfer, C. P. "Improving Organizational Communication Through Long-term Intergroup Intervention." *Journal of Applied Behavioral Science, 13* (1977): 193–210.

Argyris, C. "Diagnosing Defenses Against the Outsider." *Journal of Social Issues, 8* (3) (1952): 24–34.

Argyris, C. *Intervention Theory and Method.* Reading, MA: Addison-Wesley, 1970.

Argyris, C., & Schon, D. A. *Organizational Learning: A Theory of Action Perspective.* Reading, MA: Addison-Wesley, 1978.

Barnes, L. B. "Organizational Change and Field Experiment Methods." In *Methods of Organizational Research,* pp. 57–111. Edited by V. H. Vroom. Pittsburgh: University of Pittsburgh Press, 1967.

Beckhard, R. *Organization Development: Strategies and Models.* Reading, MA: Addison-Wesley, 1969.

Bennis, W. G. *Changing Organizations.* New York: McGraw-Hill, 1966.

Bennis, W. G. *Organization Development: Its Nature, Origins, and Prospects.* Reading, MA: Addison-Wesley, 1969.

Blake, R. R., Mouton, J. S., & Sloma, R. L. "The Union-Management Intergroup Laboratory: Strategy for Resolving Intergroup Conflict." *Journal of Applied Behavioral Science, 1* (1965): 25–57.

Bowers, D. G., & Franklin, J. L. *Survey-Guided Development: Data Based Organizational Change.* La Jolla, CA: University Associates, 1977.

Burke, W. W. "Organization Development in Transition." *Journal of Applied Behavioral Science, 12* (1976): 22–43.

Burke, W. W., & Goodstein, L. D., (Eds.) *Trends & Issues in OD: Current Theory and Practice.* San Diego, CA: University Associates, 1980.

Cammann, C., Fichman, M., Jenkins, G. D., Jr., & Klesh, J. R. "Assessing the Attitudes and Perceptions of Organizational Members." In *Assessing Organizational Change: A Guide to Methods, Measures, and Practices,* pp. 71–138. Edited by S. E. Seashore, E. E. Lawler III, P. H. Mirvis & C. Cammann. New York: Wiley, 1983.

Campbell, D. T., & Stanley, J. C. *Experimental and Quasi-Experimental Designs for Research.* Chicago: Rand McNally, 1963.

Campbell, J. P. "Psychometric Theory." In *Handbook of Industrial and Organizational Psychology,* pp. 185–222. Edited by M. D. Dunnette. Chicago: Rand McNally, 1983.

Coch, L., & French, J. R. P., Jr. "Overcoming Resistance to Change." *Human Relations, 1* (1948): 512–532.

Colligan, M. J., Smith, M. J., & Hurrell, J. J. Jr. "Occupational Incidence Rates of Mental Health Disorders." *Journal of Human Stress, 3* (1977): 34–39.

Cook, T. D., and Campbell, D. T. "The Design and Conduct of Quasi-Experiments and True Experiments in Field Settings." In *Handbook of Industrial and Organizational Psychology,* pp. 223–326. Edited by M. D. Dunnette. Chicago: Rand McNally, 1983.

Cummings, T. G., & Molloy, E. S. *Improving Productivity and the Quality of Work Life.* New York: Praeger, 1977.

Davis, L. E., & Cherns, A. B., eds. *The Quality of Working Life,* Vol. 1. New York: Free Press, 1975.

Deutsch, M. *The Resolution of Conflict: Constructive and Destructive Processes.* New Haven: Yale University Press, 1973.

Drexler, J. A., Jr., & Lawler, E. E. III "A Union-Management Cooperative Project to Improve the Quality of Work Life." *Journal of Applied Behavioral Science, 13* (1977): 373–387.

Duckles, M. M., Duckles, R., & Maccoby, M. "The Process of Change at Bolivar." *Journal of Applied Behavioral Science, 13* (1977): 387–399.

Dworkin, J. B., Extejt, M. M., & Demming, S. R. "Unionism in Hospitals, or What's Happened Since PL 93–360?" *Health Care Management Review, 5* (1980): 75–81.

Filley, A. C. *Interpersonal Conflict Resolution.* Glenview, IL: Scott, Foresman & Co., 1975.

Fox, E., & Urwick, L. *Dynamic Administration.* New York: Pitman, 1973.

French, W. L., & Bell, C. H., Jr. *Organization Development.* 2nd ed. Englewood Cliffs, NJ: Prentice-Hall, 1978.

Friedlander, F., & Brown, L. D. "Organization Development." In *Annual Review of Psychology,* Vol. 25, pp. 313–341. Edited by M. R. Rosenzweig & L. W. Porter. Palo Alto: Annual Reviews Inc., 1974.

Georgopoulos, B. S. *Organization Research on Health Institutions.* Ann Arbor, MI: Institute for Social Research, 1972.

Georgopoulos, B. S., & Mann, F. C. *The Community General Hospital.* New York: Macmillan, 1962.

Goldsmith, S. B. *Health Care Management: Perspectives for Today.* Rockville, MD: Aspen Systems Corp., 1981.

Goodman, P. S., & Dean, J. W., Jr. "Creating Long-term Organizational Change." In *Change in Organizations,* pp. 226–279. Edited by P. S. Goodman and Associates. San Francisco: Jossey-Bass, 1982.

Gordon, G., & Morse, E. V. "Evaluation Research: A Critical Review." *The Annual Review of Sociology, 1* (1975): 339–361.

Guest, R. H. "The Role of the Doctor in Institutional Management." In *Organization Research on Health Institutions,* pp. 283–300. Edited by B. S. Georgopoulos. Ann Arbor, MI: Institute for Social Research, 1972.

Hackman, J. R., & Suttle, J. L. *Improving Life at Work: Behavioral Science Approaches to Organizational Change.* Santa Monica, CA: Goodyear, 1977.

Hanlon, M. D. "Observational Methods in Organizational Assessment." In *Organizational Assessment: Perspectives on the Measurement of Organizational Behavior and the Quality of Work Life,* pp. 349–371. Edited by E. E. Lawler, III, D. A. Nadler, & C. Cammann. New York: Wiley, 1980.

Hanlon, M. D. "Unions, Productivity, and the New Industrial Relations: Strategic Considerations." *Interfaces: An International Journal of The Institute of Management Sciences and the Operations Research Society of America* (forthcoming, 1985).

Haussmann, R. K. D., Hegyvary, S. T., & Newman, J. F. *Monitoring Quality of Nursing Care, Part II: Assessment and Study of Correlates.* U.S. Department of Health, Education & Welfare, July, 1978.

Hegyvary, S. T., & Haussmann, R. K. D. "Monitoring Nursing Care Quality." *Journal of Nursing Administration, 9* (November, 1976): 3–9.

Jelinek, R. C., Haussmann, R. K. D., Hegyvary, S. T., & Newman, J. F. *A Methodology for Measuring Quality of Nursing Care.* U.S. Department of Health, Education & Welfare, January, 1974.

Kahn, R. L. et al. *Organizational Stress: Studies in Role Conflict and Ambiguity.* New York: Wiley, 1964.

Katz, D., & Kahn, R. L. *The Social Psychology of Organizations.* New York: Wiley, 1966.

Katz, H. C., Kochan, T. A., & Gobeille, K. R. "Industrial Relations Performance, Economic Performance and Quality of Working Life Efforts: An Inter-plant Analysis." Working Paper, Sloan School of Management, MIT, April, 1983.

Klein, S. M., Kraut, A. I., & Wolfson, A. "Employee Reactions to Attitude Survey Feedback: A Study of the Impact of Structure and Process." *Administrative Science Quarterly, 16* (1971): 497–514.

Kochan, T. A., & Dyer, L. "A Model of Organizational Change in the Context of Union-Management Relations." *Journal of Applied Behavioral Science, 12* (1976): 59–78.

Kochan, T. A., & McKersie, R. B. "Collective Bargaining—Pressures for Change." *Sloan Management Review* (Summer 1983): 59–65.

Kornhauser, A. W. *Mental Health of the Industrial Worker: A Detroit Study.* New York: Wiley, 1965.

Lawler, E. E. III. "Adaptive Experiments: An Approach to Organizational Behavior Research." *Academy of Management Review, 2* (1977): 576–585.

Lawler, E. E. III. "Increasing Worker Involvement to Enhance Organizational Effectiveness." In *Change in Organizations,* pp. 280–315. Edited by P. S. Goodman & Associates. San Francisco: Jossey-Bass, 1982.

Lawler, E. E. III. "Measuring the Quality of Working Life: The Why and How of It." In *The Quality of Working Life,* Vol. 1, pp. 123–133. Edited by L. E. Davis & A. B. Cherns. New York: Free Press, 1975.

Lawler, E. E. III. *Motivation in Work Organizations.* Monterey, CA: Brooks/Cole, 1973.

Lawler, E. E. III, Nadler, D. A., & Cammann, C. *Organizational Assessment: Perspectives on the Measurement of Organizational Behavior and the Quality of Working Life.* New York: Wiley, 1980.

Lawler, E. E. III, Nadler, D. A., & Mirvis, P. H. "Organizational Change and the Conduct of Assessment Research." In *Assessing Organizational Change: A Guide to Methods,*

Measures, and Practices, pp. 19–47. Edited by S. E. Seashore, E. E. Lawler III, P. H. Mirvis, & C. Cammann. New York: Wiley, 1983.

Likert, R., & Likert, J. G. *New Ways of Managing Conflict.* New York: McGraw-Hill, 1976.

Lesieur, F. G. *The Scanlon Plan: A Frontier in Labor-Management Cooperation.* Cambridge, MA: MIT Press, 1958.

Levinson, H., Price, C. R., Mundell, K. S., Mandl, H. J., & Solley, C. M., *Men, Management and Mental Health.* Cambridge: Harvard University Press, 1962.

Lewicki, R. J., & Alderfer, C. P. "The Tensions Between Research and Intervention in Intergroup Conflict." *Journal of Applied Behavioral Science, 9* (1973): 424–449.

Macy, B. A., & Mirvis, P. H. "Assessing Rates and Costs of Individual Work Behaviors." In *Assessing Organizational Change: A Guide to Methods, Measures, and Practices,* pp. 139–176. Edited by S. E. Seashore, E. E. Lawler III, P. H. Mirvis & C. Cammann. New York: Wiley, 1983.

Mechanic, D. *Medical Sociology.* 2nd ed. New York: Free Press, 1978.

Mirvis, P. H., & Berg, D. N. *Failures in Organization Development and Change: Cases and Essays for Learning.* New York: Wiley, 1977.

Moses, E., & Roth, A. "What Do Statistics Reveal about the Nation's Nurses?" *American journal of Nursing, 79* (1979): 1745–56.

Nadler, D. A. *Feedback and Organization Development: Using Data Based Methods.* Reading, MA: Addison-Wesley, 1977.

Nadler, D. A. "Hospitals, Organized Labor and Quality of Work: An Intervention Case Study." *Journal of Applied Behavioral Science, 14* (1978): 366–381.

Nadler, D. A., Hackman, J. R., & Lawler, E. E. III. *Managing Organizational Behavior.* Boston: Little, Brown and Company, 1979.

Nadler, D. A., Hanlon, M. D., & Lawler, E. E. III. "Factors Influencing the Success of Labor-Management Quality of Work Life Projects." *Journal of Occupational Behaviour, 1* (1980), 53–67.

Nadler, D. A., Jenkins, G. D., Mirvis, P. H., & Macy, B. A. "A Research Design and Measurement Package for the Assessment of Quality of Work Interventions." *Proceedings of the 35th Annual Meeting of the Academy of Management* (1975): 360–362.

Nadler, D. A., Perkins, D. N. T., & Hanlon, M. D. "The Observation of Organizational Behavior: A Structured Naturalistic Approach." In *Assessing Organizational Change: A Guide to Methods, Measures, and Practices,* pp. 331–352. Edited by S. E. Seashore, E. E. Lawler III, P. H. Mirvis, & C. Cammann. New York: Wiley, 1983.

Nadler, D. A., & Tichy, N. M. "The Limitations of Traditional Intervention Technologies in Health Care Organizations." In *Organizational Development in Health Care Organizations,* pp. 359–378. Edited by N. Margulies, & J. Adams. Reading, MA: Addison-Wesley, 1980.

Nadler, D. A., & Tushman, M. L. "A Diagnostic Model for Organizational Behavior." In *Perspectives on Behavior in Organizations,* pp. 85–98. Edited by J. R. Hackman, E. E. Lawler III, & L. W. Porter. New York: McGraw-Hill, 1977.

Nieva, V. F., & Perkins, D. N. T. "The Organizational Assessment Role: Issues and Dilemmas." In *Organizational Assessment: Perspectives on the Measurement of Organizational Behavior and the Quality of Work Life,* pp. 569–581. Edited by E. E. Lawler III, D. A. Nadler, & C. Cammann. New York: Wiley, 1980.

Nunnally, J. C. *Psychometric Theory.* New York: McGraw-Hill, 1978.

Perkins, D. N. T., Nieva, V. F., & Lawler, E. E. III. *Managing Creation: The Challenge of Building a New Organization.* New York: Wiley, 1983.

Perrow, C. "Goals and Power Structures: A Historical Case Study." In *The Hospital in Modern Society,* pp. 112–146. Edited by E. Freidson. New York: Free Press, 1963.

Sashkin, M., Morris, W. C., & Horst, L. "A Comparison of Social and Organizational Change Models: Information Flow and Data Use Processes." *Psychological Review, 80* (1973): 510–526.

Schatzman, L., & Strauss, A. L. *Field Research: Strategies for a Natural Sociology.* Englewood Cliffs, NJ: Prentice-Hall, 1973.

Schein, E. H. "The Mechanisms of Change." In *The Planning of Change,* 2nd ed., pp. 98–107. Edited by W. G. Bennis, K. D. Benne, & R. Chin. New York: Holt, Rinehart & Winston, 1969.

Seashore, S. E. "Field Experiments with Formal Organizations." *Human Organization, 23* (1964): 164–170.

Seashore, S. E. "Issues in Assessing Organizational Change." In *Assessing Organizational Change: A Guide to Methods, Measures, and Practices,* pp. 49–66. Edited by S. E. Seashore, E. E. Lawler III, P. H. Mirvis, & C. Cammann. New York: Wiley, 1983.

Sexton, P. C. *The New Nightingales: Hospital Workers, Unions, New Women's Issues.* New York: Enquiry Press, 1982.

Siegel, I. H., & Weinberg, E. *Labor-Management Cooperation: The American Experience.* Kalamzoo, MI: The W. E. Upjohn Institute for Employment Research, 1982.

Starr, P. *The Social Transformation of American Medicine: The Rise of a Soverign Profession and the Making of a Vast Industry.* New York: Basic Books, 1982.

Thomas, K. "Conflict and Conflict Management." In *Handbook of Industrial and Organizational Psychology,* pp. 889–935. Edited by M. D. Dunnette. Chicago: Rand McNally, 1983.

Toch, H., & Grant, J. D. *Reforming Human Services: Change Through Participation.* Beverly Hills, CA: Sage Publications, 1982.

Tushman, M. L., & Nadler, D. A. "Information Processing as an Integrating Concept in Organizational Design." *Academy of Management Review, 3* (1978): 613–624.

U.S. Department of Health, Education & Welfare. *Work in America.* Cambridge, MA: MIT Press, 1973.

Vroom, V. H. *Work and Motivation.* New York: Wiley, 1964.

Walton, R. D. "The Diffusion of New Work Structures: Explaining Why Success Didn't Take." In *Failures in Organizational Development and Change: Cases and Essays for Learning,* pp. 243–261. Edited by P. H. Mirvis & D. N. Berg. New York: Wiley, 1977.

Walton, R. E., & McKersie, R. B. *A Behavioral Theory of Labor Negotiations.* New York: McGraw-Hill, 1965.

Walton, R. E. *Interpersonal Peacemaking: Confrontations and Third-Party Consultation.* Reading, MA: Addison-Wesley, 1969.

Warr, P. B., & Wall, T. *Work and Well-Being.* Baltimore: Penguin Books, 1976.

Weick, C. E. "Repunctuating the Problem." In *New Perspectives in Organizational Effectiveness,* pp. 193–225. Edited by P. S. Goodman, J. M. Pennings, and Associates. San Francisco: Josey-Bass, 1977.

Weisbord, M. R. "Why Organization Development Hasn't Worked (So Far) in Medical Centers." *Health Care Management Review, 1* (1976): 17–28.

Weisbord, M. R., & Goodstein, L., eds. "Toward Healthier Medical Systems: Can We Learn From Experience?" *Journal of Applied Behavioral Science, 14* (1978): 263–264.

Zand, D. E. "Collateral Organization: A New Change Strategy." *Journal of Applied Behavioral Science, 10* (1974): 63–89.

Author Index

Subject Index

Absenteeism, 164, 181, 184-185
Action research, 14
American Center for the Quality of
Working Life, 5, 13. *See also*
National Quality of Work
Center
Assessment:
  of Barnard 5 subproject, 118-121,
    175, 178-196
  of Barnard training program, 193-
    195
  of clinical services subproject, 168-
    169, 175, 200-215
  of communication network sub-
    project, 170, 175, 196-198
  of consultants' strategy, 118-122,
    150-154
  of early stages of QWL program, 63-
    64, 220-222
  of first consultant group, 82-87, 222
  of organization mirroring subproject,
    175, 215-217
  problems of, 156-157, 160-163,
    173-174
  of project outcome determinants,
    220-227
  of second consultant group, 106-
    107, 222
  strategy for, 158-160, 163-170, 173-
    177

  unresolved issues in, 170-172

Barnard 5 subproject:
  assessment of, 118-121, 175, 178-
    196
  history of, 75-81, 92-107, 124-
    126
Board of trustees, 26-28

Clinical services subproject:
  assessment of, 168-169, 175, 200-
    215
  history of, 111-114, 131-133, 198-
    200
Collective bargaining, 16
Communication network
    subproject:
  assessment of, 170, 175, 196-198
  history of, 129-131
Consultants:
  dismissal of first consultant team,
    81-82
  organizational development plan of,
    94, 229-232
  role of, 20-22
  selection of first consultant team,
    58-64
  selection of second consultant team,
    89-92
  strategy of, 109-118, 161

247

Quality of work life (QWL):
  concerns about, 17-18
  definition of, 11-12
Quality of Work Life Intervention
  Design, 11, 13-23

Research, design of, 22, 158-170.
  See also Assessment, strategy for
Researchers, role of, 22, 170-172

Staff conferences, 99-100, 120-121,
  125
State Nurses' Association, 29, 32, 45,

50-54, 102, 104
Structured naturalistic observation,
  190, 213, 216
Survey feedback, 131-133, 201-210,
  213-214

Training program (Barnard):
  assessment of, 122, 193-195
  description of, 115-118, 126-129

Underbounded systems, 41-42
Unions, involvement in QWL, vii-viii,
  6-7, 226-227